RESEARCH AND ETHICS
FOR THE MEDICAL PROFESSION

RESEARCH AND ETHICS FOR THE MEDICAL PROFESSION

First Edition

J M Albareeq

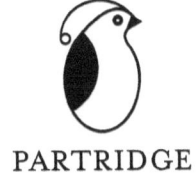

PARTRIDGE

Copyright © 2017 by Jaffar M Albareeq.

ISBN: Softcover   978-1-5437-4103-2
          eBook   978-1-5437-4102-5

All rights reserved. No part of this book may be used or reproduced by any means, graphic, electronic, or mechanical, including photocopying, recording, taping or by any information storage retrieval system without the written permission of the author except in the case of brief quotations embodied in critical articles and reviews.

Because of the dynamic nature of the Internet, any web addresses or links contained in this book may have changed since publication and may no longer be valid. The views expressed in this work are solely those of the author and do not necessarily reflect the views of the publisher, and the publisher hereby disclaims any responsibility for them.

Print information available on the last page.

To order additional copies of this book, contact
Toll Free 800 101 2657 (Singapore)
Toll Free 1 800 81 7340 (Malaysia)
orders.singapore@partridgepublishing.com

www.partridgepublishing.com/singapore

CONTENTS AT GLANCE

1. Introduction 1
2. Ethics of the Medical Profession 13
3. Ethics and the Law 67
4. Consent 79
5. Teaching Ethics to Medical Students and Residents 91
6. End-of-Life Care Policy 101
7. Ethical Standards in Psychiatric Practice 121
8. Ethical Perspectives in Oncology Practice 137
9. Ethics of Gastrointestinal Endoscopy 155
10. Ethics in Nursing and the Nursing Process 171
11. The Ethics of Hyperbaric Oxygen Therapy 187
12. Ethics in the Clinical Laboratory 193
13. Vision of the Future King Hamad Research Center 207
14. Basic Principles of the Belmont Report[1] 211

CONTRIBUTORS

Dr. Jaffar Albareeq, DLO, RCS, RCP
Consultant ENT Surgeon
Director of Ethics and Research Committee
Chairman of CME and Morbidity Committees
Chief Editor of Bahrain Medical Bulletin
King Hamad University Hospital

Dr. Adel Abdul Aal, MD, MSc, FCHM
Consultant and Head
Hyperbaric Oxygen Therapy and Wound Care
King Hamad University Hospital

Dr. Hamdy Hasan Abozenah, MD, PhD
Consultant Nephrologist
King Hamad University Hospital
Associate Professor
Royal College of Surgeons in Ireland, Medical University of Bahrain (RCSI-MUB)

Dr. Fairouz Alhourani, PhD, CBAHI
Director of Nursing
King Hamad University Hospital

Dr. Dalal Alromaihi, MD
Consultant Endocrinologist
King Hamad University Hospital
Senior Clinical Lecturer
RCSI-MUB, Bahrain

Major Abdullah Alsowaidi, LLB, Bch, MS, MSC
Director of Legal Affairs
King Hamad University Hospital
Senior Lecturer
University College of Bahrain

Dr. Suhail Baithun, MBCHB, FRCPath
Consultant Histopathologist
Senior Clinical Lecturer
RCSI-MUB, Bahrain

Dr. Martin Corbally, MCh, FRCSI, FRCSEd, FRCS, MRCPI, CCST
Chief of Medical Staff
Consultant Pediatric Surgeon (Neonatal, Hepatobiliary and Oncology)
King Hamad University Hospital
Professor and Head of the Department of Surgery, RCSI Bahrain

Dr. Elias Fadel, MD
Consultant Hematologist - Oncologist
Director of Oncology Center
King Hamad University Hospital
Senior Lecturer
RCSI-MUB, Bahrain

Dr. Omar Sharif, MD
Consultant Gastroenterologist
King Hamad University Hospital
Senior Clinical Lecturer
RCSI-MUB, Bahrain

Ms. Sharon Skowronski, RN
Nursing Manager
King Hamad University Hospital

Dr. Eamon Tierney, BAO, FFARCSI, FJFICMI
Associate Professor of Surgery
RCSI-MUB, Bahrain
Director of ICU and Consultant Intensivist/Anesthetist
King Hamad University Hospital

INTRODUCTION

Martin T. Corbally

The publication of this book marks the culmination of an ambition to improve and enhance our understanding of ethics in the key areas of research and clinical practice. As practicing physicians, we are all aware of the requirement for consistent ethical practice, both in research and clinical medicine. Doctors are the ultimate advocates for patients and the health and welfare of our fellow man; however, they often find themselves in difficulty with current issues of informed consent, inter-professional relationships, maintenance of patient confidentiality and the requirements for good clinical practice (GCP) in research.

Dr. Jaffar Albareeq, who generated the idea for this book, resourced the various contributing editors and maintained the correct resilience to see it to publication, is to be congratulated on providing this reference text, which is both practical and theoretical in its objective to enhance our practical understanding of this dynamic area. The book also underscores the benefits and requirements of research and its interface with research involving human subjects.

The book contains chapters from practicing doctors and nurses who are familiar with the daily ethical dilemmas that are the norm of clinical engagement. Ethical issues and debates surrounding them have been with us since the time of Hippocrates, and while it is relatively easy to be complacent with these matters or simply refer the issue to an ethics committee, it not only behooves the practicing clinician and nurse to develop a self-driven philosophy that facilitates good clinical practice, but also acknowledges ethics as a fluid dynamic that changes with time, jurisdiction and the individual patient.

The contributing editors have a wealth of individual experience and a deep insight into local circumstances that may vary the unique interpretation of any ethical dilemma. The book is also intended to report and encourage our efforts to engage in research, both laboratory and clinical. In many areas, the focus is to emphasize the current and recommended practice at King Hamad University Hospital, which despite its infancy, has developed international standards in health care practice, ethics and research.

Thirteen individual experts have contributed 13 chapters to this book. In the first chapter, Dr. Jaffar Albareeq leads a discussion on "Ethics of the Medical Profession." It details the general duties of a doctor and what it means to be a doctor in the modern world. It also includes the importance of ethical relationships with colleagues and the sanctity of the doctor-patient relationship. Dr. Jaffar goes to some lengths to describe the appropriate doctor-to-doctor behavior and is particularly cautionary about openly criticizing the practice of another physician.

Various problems may arise in practice because of poor ethical behavior. That undermines the society's confidence, not only in the doctor who has a natural right to a good reputation, but also in the profession as a whole and it serves an invalid purpose and promotes the unacceptable practice. Disrespectful behavior towards another doctor is never acceptable and practitioners must act professionally at all times. The chapter also highlights certain areas that have been blurred recently, such as advertising and fraud. The profession needs to maintain a careful vigil in these areas and ensure compliance.

This first chapter is, in essence, a practical guide to the ethics of everyday clinical practice. It deals extensively with the value of clinical research and importantly emphasizes the requirements for good clinical practice, especially when involving human subjects.

The components of modern versions of the Hippocratic Oath, such as the Geneva Declaration of the World Medical Association, clearly states the doctor's ethical responsibility in not engaging in a practice that renders a patient physically or mentally vulnerable in any way. Practice contrary to the laws of the Kingdom of Bahrain, such as abortion and sterilization are also addressed later in the book. The book closes with a notable summary of the Belmont Report which functions as the KHUH reference for all research performed. It enshrines respect for the research subject, beneficence in research, confidentiality, informed consent and the right of the research subject to withdraw consent at any time.

The theme of the psychiatric chapter details the vulnerability of the patient in the doctor-patient relationship and how this must never be abused. The Madrid Declaration on Ethical Standards for Psychiatric Practice deals with the ethical perspective in psychiatry. Of all clinical specialties, psychiatry has perhaps the greatest insight into the vulnerability of the patients, potential abuse of these patients and how the profession must safeguard against this potential. Medicine is both an art and science, a statement relevant to modern practice where we often forget that we are here not just to treat the disease, but the patient as a whole. The Madrid Declaration explores many sensitive issues, such as euthanasia, which while accepted as a therapeutic option in some European countries, is illegal in all Middle Eastern countries, such as Bahrain. The discussion addresses the role of the psychiatrist in this morally complex area and also refers to legal cases, genetic research, dementia and consent. Some of these themes are discussed later in the book. One of the key messages, however, is that the psychiatrist plays an invaluable and expert role in assessing a patient's understanding in the pivotal area of informed consent, and crucially when a patient wishes to decline consent.

Professor Eamon Tierney, Associate Professor of Surgery at the Royal College of Surgeons in Ireland, Bahrain, and Consultant Intensivist-Anesthetist and Director of ICU at King Hamad University Hospital, provides a general view of end-of-life care and the decision making process that allows a patient, legal guardian and relatives come to terms with a decision to allow their loved one exit this life with dignity and compassion. The subject is complex, but resonates well with the ICU staff and those involved in areas where this is common, such as Oncology. It is also addressed later by Nurse Sharon Skowronski, Nursing Manager and Dr. Elias Fadel, Consultant Hematologist-Oncologist at King Hamad University Hospital. End-of-life care is primarily indicated in cases where there is no cure available or when medical efforts are futile and aim to allow death with dignity. It includes concepts such as "Do Not Resuscitate (DNR)", which are open to constant review and amendment as circumstances change. It is often quoted that this concept is not acceptable in the Islamic faith; however, there are numerous 'fatwas' which indicate that it is an acceptable strategy in cases where there is no hope. The decision must be confirmed by three physicians.

The process of Consent and Informed Consent and how it has evolved over time to what it is today was reviewed in a chapter on its own. This contribution comes from me, Professor Martin Corbally, Consultant Pediatric Surgeon and Chief of Staff at King Hamad University Hospital and Professor of Surgery at the Royal College of Surgeons in Ireland, Bahrain. The chapter attempts to resolve the uncertainty that many doctors experience as to how much information a patient should be given to obtain valid consent. It is very clear that consent is a necessary component of all treatments. It is not always necessary to list each and every potential complication, which would be a daunting task and likely to instill unnecessary anxiety in the patient. The modern approach dictates that the information given is what a reasonable patient would wish to know before giving their consent to a procedure. Fortunately, most patients are reasonable, and this approach avoids the overly paternalistic approach of the reasonable doctor. The latter would be well advised to seek input from other physicians/professionals when dealing with an unreasonable patient as the doctor could well be accused of assault if the agreed procedure is not fully understood by the patient. Consent for a procedure does not excuse or render the physician immune from criticism or censorship in the event of complications, but merely allows the attending care team permission to carry out the procedure or test. Essentially, a reasonable patient needs to know about a rare risk if it is substantial and may affect the quality of the patient's life.

Many of the examples listed in this chapter are landmark cases in the evolution of procedural consent, from no explanation of risk to the legal requirement for full disclosure. While cultural concerns would arise from time to time, there could be little doubt that every significant risk must be detailed at the time of consent. That applies if the risk is very rare, such as 1 in 15,000. Consent is a two-way dynamic where the doctor imparts information in clear language, and the patient has the right and time to clarify any detail of concern. The chapter highlights difficult areas in consent, such as in minors, where the International Guidelines state that while not legally necessary, it is best to include them in the discussion and consent in situations of questionable mental capacity. In this situation, consent may be given by a legal guardian, but it should be noted that, in such cases, it is the ability of the patient to understand the suggested treatment plan and the consequences of refusal of treatment.

Gastroenterology chapter is a contribution from Dr. Omar Sharif, Consultant Gastroenterologist, Deputy Chief of Staff at King Hamad University Hospital and Senior Lecturer in Medicine at the Royal College of Surgeons in Ireland, Bahrain. This chapter focuses on the areas of consent for gastrointestinal procedures and the potential complications from these varied procedures. Dr. Sharif makes the point that when a recognized complication occurs, such as perforation during colonoscopy, the physician would not be liable provided the consent has clearly detailed this as a possible risk. Consent is an issue that requires focused attention as detailed by Dr. Sharif. The ethics of screening procedures in the elderly are also dealt with and clearly there is a moral obligation to consider the appropriateness of such screening interventions in those at the extreme of life. Patients in this age group are of course ethically entitled to the same standards of care, but the United States Preventive Screening Task Force has recommended that patients over 85 years of age are not subject to routine screening and that patients between 75 and 85 should not undergo routine screening unless there are specific indications.

Doctor Sharif also explores the confusing and challenging issue of gastrostomy feeding in the elderly patient. While artificial feeding is a medical treatment, it is also true that like all medical treatments, it must be considered with reference to the individual patient. Society may consider artificial feeding as a human right, but it is not always wise or moral to provide that. Patients with end-stage disease, advanced dementia, should not undergo gastrostomy placement, as end-of-life care does not include such attempts at prolongation of life, and adjustments of medications and nutritional formula may otherwise facilitate normal enteral feeding. Patients who have the potential for prolonged survival and are nasogastric tube-fed should always be considered for alternative feeding regimens.

The Pathology and Laboratory Chapter is provided by Dr. Suhail Baithun, Consultant Histopathologist at King Hamad University Hospital, Senior Lecturer at the Royal College of Surgeons in Ireland, Bahrain and former Associate Professor at the Royal London Hospital, United Kingdom. This chapter reviews the ethical requirements of practice from the clinical laboratory. It is not unusual to forget or minimize the extreme importance of the clinical laboratory and its impact on patient management. He details the duty of the laboratory to medical colleagues and the patient in preserving the dignity of the profession and maintaining a reputation of honesty, respect, integrity and reliability. It preserves a duty to provide accurate information while guarding patient confidentiality and training successive medical and technical staff. At all times, the patient has the right to access information held about them in the clinical laboratory; however, such information must be adequately stored as confidentiality is of the utmost importance. Dr. Suhail makes a valuable comment on the geographical and cultural difficulties that exist due to the general reluctance to perform an autopsy and highlights the benefits of "virtual autopsy" to provide more detail. Finally, he makes a plea that like the Hippocratic Oath, all technical medical laboratory staff should follow the lead of the American Society for Clinical Laboratory Science and take an appropriate pledge to provide high-quality care.

The chapter on Medical Ethics to Undergraduate Students addresses the real need for medical schools to teach such an important topic. The chapter is the contribution of Dr. Dalal Alromaihi, Consultant Endocrinologist at King Hamad University Hospital and Senior Lecturer at the Royal College of Surgeons in Ireland, Bahrain. Dr. Dalal is the recipient of the Award for Humanism from the Arnold P. Gold – Gold Humanism Honor Society in 2009 and the Role Model Award for Medical Students from Wayne State University, Detroit, Michigan.

Considering that medicine is a moral profession, it is not possible to separate good clinical practice from professional and ethical behavior. Dr. Dalal makes a cogent argument for the manner in which ethics is taught to medical students, stating that case-based scenarios led by dedicated and experienced clinicians are more productive than formal classroom sessions. Mentorship, encouragement and student engagement in relevant ethical dilemmas should be the mainstay of ethical undergraduate teaching, which is increasingly part of the undergraduate medical curriculum. Role-playing and feedback are crucial to undergraduate progression to preserve the unique idealism of the undergraduate and to aid in the development of ethical maturity. There could be little doubt that ethical education has been missing from the curricula of many medical schools; however, it is equally as important as clinical education.

Hyperbaric Oxygen Therapy Chapter is written by Dr. Adel Abdul Aal, Director and Consultant in Charge of the Hyperbaric Oxygen Therapy (HBOT) Unit at King Hamad University Hospital, Bahrain. Dr. Adel has added responsibility in the oversight of wound management in conjunction with other KHUH clinicians. As a relatively new therapy, HBOT has had to define its unique set of ethical guidelines that govern the use of this therapy in as yet fully defined areas. Similar to any therapy, both established and innovative, it is crucial not only that all referring physicians are aware of the indications for such treatment, but also that the providers understand and apply a risk-benefit solution to each referral. Dr. Adel develops a useful platform to facilitate its use even in situations where the therapy is unproven. It includes full informed consent, therapy delivered by fully qualified clinicians and the development of a full database that would contribute to research and perhaps develop solid conclusions to the benefits of this novel therapy.

The chapter provided by Major Abdulla Alsowaidi, Director of Legal Affairs, King Hamad University Hospital and Senior Lecturer, University College of Bahrain seeks to review the interface between the law of the land and medical ethics. While it is interesting to believe that ethics and the law must always agree or at least reach the same conclusion, it is clear from this chapter that the law progresses at a slower pace than that of ethical guidelines. From a societal perspective, slow changes in the law are protective to the fabric of society, yet the lag time between the law and ethics often creates a logistical difficulty for clinicians. Major Abdulla highlights areas of Bahrain law that are in need of modernization to bring them in line with international standards, such as abortion and end-of-life care. It is clear that the medical profession must always act as the patient's advocate, but must always be within the boundaries of the law to avoid conflict with the legislature. Ethical principles must be enshrined in legislation in so far as possible.

The chapter ends with a discussion on medical indemnity, which is of equal importance to the practicing doctor and is currently undergoing change in Bahrain. Society is subject to multiple influences, not all of which are realistic. It is unreasonable to expect that every intervention would produce a positive outcome; however, the patient has the right to expect a high standard of care. While recognizing that complications could and do occur, it is important that the physician accepts the necessity for fully informed consent and deals with untoward events openly and honestly. Each medical institution is ethically obliged to ensure that it adheres to the legal requirements as laid down by the National Health Regulatory Authority (NHRA Bahrain) and that significant negative outcomes are reported. The primary goal of reportage is to ensure that lessons are learned and not repeated.

The chapter on Nursing is the contribution by Dr. Fairouz Alhourani, Director of Nursing and Sharon Skowronski, Nursing Manager at King Hamad University Hospital. The chapter deals with important topics of ethics in nursing and the nursing process. The role of the nurse in the formulation of ethical practice is often overlooked; yet, the moral and ethical backdrop for many ethical discussions occur at this level.

Arguably, nurses occupy a pivotal position between the patient and the clinical team; hence, the moral barometer of ethical decisions as they apply to their patient. The authors address this and pointed out that it may cause stress to the nurse when a clinical decision is not clear. It may arise when the nurse, while caring for the overall needs of the patient, is unable to decide what is the most medically appropriate and best treatment for the patient or by extrapolation the limitations of any planned intervention. The nurse has an equal duty to preserve patient confidence and while the authors suggest that the moral basis of confidentiality is unclear, it indicates a greater role for team discussions to overcome these traditional barriers. Rather than focusing solely on a patient cure, the nurse code of practice embraces support and nurturing of the patient in a more holistic sense. It is much more advanced and inclusive than a narrow view of the nurse as prevalent 50 years ago.

The chapter on Ethics in Oncological Practice is contributed by Dr. Elias Fadel, Consultant Hematologist-Oncologist and Director of the new National Oncology Centre at King Hamad University Hospital. The chapter leads with the important topic of breaking bad news, which is of great significance in oncology where oncologists are regularly called to impart a difficult diagnosis. Clear guidelines are enumerated as to how this news is to be conveyed. This is derived from a variety of sources and protocols of communication, but it is evident that oncologists are the most qualified to do so. As in every medical interaction, informed consent is a vital part of the process, and this especially applies to oncological diagnosis and treatment. It is evident and ethical that all patients have the right to know their diagnosis and be given a realistic estimate of the risk of complications, the rate of cure and the likelihood of disease progression.

While this is the norm in Western society, it is not always the case in Bahrain or the Middle East. That creates tension between doctor and patient and it is well addressed by Dr. Fadel. The chapter also deals with "do not resuscitate concept" which is of even greater relevance in oncology where inevitably, some patients would die of their disease. The subject has been discussed in a previous chapter in a general sense, but here, it is specifically directed towards patients dying with cancer. Dr. Fadel deals empathetically and compassionately with the problem, the cultural difficulties that could surround this diagnosis and the importance of accepting the patient's beliefs, which may be at variance with that of the caregiver.

CONCLUSION

This seminal work "Research and Ethics for the Medical Profession" shares a common thread amongst all its contributing authors, and that the medical and nursing profession are obligated to act compassionately, honestly and with respect for the betterment of their patients. Doctors have a moral duty to act within the law of the land while recognizing that at times the legislature may lag behind the evolving and at times urgent needs of the profession. The culture of respect for one's patient is essential in the doctor-doctor relationship and preserves society's confidence in the doctor and the profession at large. Respect for the patient exists at each stage of the doctor-patient interaction as informed consent or when the patient rejects the planned procedure or requests a second opinion.

This book would provide a guide to the professional working in today's complex environment; however, the physician should always place his patient first and never be afraid to admit uncertainty or seek help.

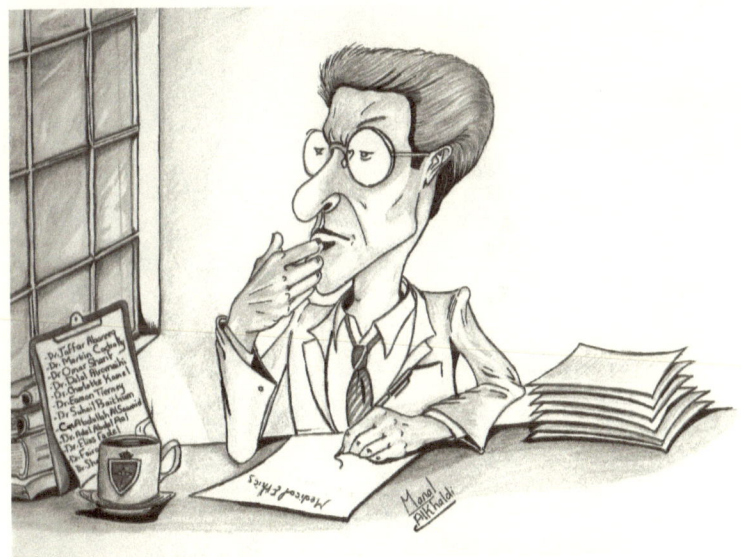

ETHICS OF THE MEDICAL PROFESSION

Jaffar M. Albareeq

Character of the Medical Profession

The profession of medicine is an ancient human, ethical and scientific activity, as old as humankind. This antiquity has been endowed with practices and qualities, compelling its practitioner to respect humanity in all conditions and states, to be a fine example in his behavior and treatment, upright in his dealing, to preserve and honor human life, to be compassionate towards his patients and to do his best in serving them.

An International Code of Medical Ethics

One of the first acts of the World Medical Association in 1948 to unite the profession throughout the world in a single brotherhood was to produce a modern restatement of the Hippocratic Oath known as the "Declaration of Geneva", and to base upon it an International Code of Medical Ethics, which applies both in times of peace and war. The Declaration of Geneva states[1]:

At the Time of Being Admitted as a Member of the Medical Profession

I solemnly pledge myself to consecrate my life to the service of humanity; I will give to my teachers the respect and gratitude which is their due;

I will practice my profession with conscience and dignity; The health of my patient will be my first consideration;

I will respect the secrets which are confided in me;

I will maintain by all the means in my power the honor and the noble traditions of the medical profession;

My colleagues will be my brothers;

I will not permit considerations of religion, nationality, race, party politics or social standing to intervene between my duty and my patient;

I will maintain the utmost respect for human life from the time of conception, even under threat; I will not use my medical knowledge contrary to the laws of humanity.

I make these promises solemnly, freely and upon my honor.

Research

King Hamad University Hospital would remain committed to encourage research and researchers in Bahrain. The aim of research is to improve people's health and quality of life. No research should be performed without the approval of the Research and Ethical Committee; some research proposals would be funded by KHUH if the budget for such department is available.

KHUH Research Committee Objectives

1. To encourage research in all fields of medicine, including medico-legal cases.
2. To provide research service for medical and allied health researchers at KHUH.
3. To work with the researcher to develop a specific aim for his research study.
4. To design research protocol for the researcher.
5. To edit research at all stages and help the researcher prepare preliminary results.
6. To help the researcher publish the research study in medical journals or books.
7. To guide the researcher through grant applications and approval.
8. To help the researcher prepare research budget.
9. To help the researcher avail resources, facilities and available support.
10. To help the researcher adhere and abide by ethical principles and guidelines for the protection of human subjects of research.
11. To help the government save millions by finding the best and most efficient way to treat any condition; the most efficient medication to be purchased for public consumption, not to forget the tremendous patient's benefits.

12. To allocate the time and funds for those clinicians interested in research rather than to depend on overstretched practitioners; therefore, the traditional excuse "lack of funds and time" would no longer be applicable.
13. To include commissioned research based on the national health priorities in Bahrain.
14. To promote and support quality research and enhance the opportunity for medical and paramedical professionals to conduct research relevant to the patients.
15. To promote national, regional and international collaborations in science and medical research for the sake of improving health.
16. To continue the search for a new field of science and medical research relevant to improving the health of patients in Bahrain with a specific focus on genetic diseases.
17. To establish a National Electronic Library for Health, which would contain a fully searchable database of all health care research conducted by Bahraini researchers, as well as provide an open access real-time resource for healthcare providers, researchers and policy makers.

Scientific research has produced substantial health benefits. It has also produced some disturbing ethical dilemmas. The public is concerned about the abuse of human subjects and animals in biomedical research. To avoid such abuse, we will work closely with the researcher to adhere to the basic principles of ethics in research[2].

Research Could Be Divided into Primary and Secondary

A. Primary

  1. Analytic
  2. Descriptive

B. Secondary

   1. Systematic review
   2. Meta-analysis
   3. Cochrane review

Types of Studies Could Be Subdivided into:

A. Descriptive, such as a community survey
B. Analytic
C. Experimental

   a. Randomized Clinical Trial
   b. Non-randomized Clinical Trial

D. Non-experimental

   a. Cohort
   b. Case-cohort
   c. Case-control
   d. Cross-sectional

The main research field should concentrate on prevention, diagnosis and treatment of common diseases in Bahrain, such as coronary heart diseases, diabetes, hereditary blood diseases and cancer.

Human Experimentation[3]

In 1964, the World Medical Association drew up a code of ethics on human experimentation. This code is known as the Declaration of Helsinki, which states the following:

"It is the mission of the doctor to safeguard the health of the people. His knowledge and conscience are dedicated to the fulfillment of this mission."

The Declaration of Geneva of the World Medical Association binds the doctor with the words: **"The health of my patient will be my first consideration"**; the International Code of Medical Ethics states that **"Any act or advice which could weaken physical or mental resistance of a human being may be used only in his interest"**. Because it is essential that the results of laboratory experiments be applied to human beings to further scientific knowledge and to help suffering humanity, the World Medical Association has prepared the following recommendations as a guide to each doctor in clinical research. It must be stressed that the standards, as drafted, are only a guide to physicians all over the world. Doctors are not relieved from criminal, civil and ethical responsibilities under the laws of their countries.

In the field of biomedical research, a fundamental distinction must be recognized between clinical research, in which the objective is essentially therapeutic and non-therapeutic research, the essential objective of which is purely scientific and without therapeutic value to the person subjected to the research.

Basic Principles of Clinical Research

1. Clinical research must conform to the moral and scientific principles that justify medical research and should be based on laboratory and animal experiments or other scientifically established facts.
2. Clinical research should be conducted only by scientifically qualified person and under the supervision of a qualified medical professional.
3. Clinical research could not legitimately be carried out unless the importance of the objective is in proportion to the inherent risk to the subject.
4. Every clinical research project should be preceded by careful assessment of inherent risks compared to foreseeable benefits to the subject.

5. Extreme caution should be exercised by the doctor in performing clinical research in which the personality of the subject is liable to be altered by drugs or experimental procedure.

Clinical Research Combined with Professional Care

During the treatment of the sick patient, the doctor must be free to use new therapeutic measures if, in his judgment, it offers hope of saving a life, re-establishing health, or alleviating suffering.

Informed consent should be obtained from the participant. In case of legal incapacity, consent should be procured from the legal guardian; in case of physical incapacity, the permission of the legal guardian replaces that of the patient.

Non-Therapeutic Clinical Research

1. In the purely scientific application of clinical research carried out on a human being, it is the duty of the doctor to remain the protector of the life and health of that person on whom clinical research is being carried out.
2. The nature, purpose, and risk of clinical research must be explained to the subject by the doctor.
3. Clinical research on a human being could not be undertaken without his free consent after he has been fully informed (informed consent); if he is legally incompetent, the consent of the legal guardian should be procured.
4. The subject of clinical research should be in such a mental, physical, and legal state as to be able to exercise his power of choice fully.
5. Consent should, as a rule, be obtained in writing. However, the responsibility for clinical research always remains with the researcher; it never falls on the subject, even after consent is obtained.

6. The investigator must respect the right of each individual to safeguard his personal integrity, especially if the subject is in a dependent relationship with the investigator.
7. At any time during clinical research, the subject or his guardian should be free to withdraw the permission for research to be continued. The investigator or the investigating team should discontinue the research if in his or their judgment may, if continued, be harmful to the individual.

Organs from Live Donors

Written consent should be obtained from the donor after a full explanation of the procedure involved and the possible consequences to the donor. Where appropriate, the donor should be advised to discuss the procedure with his or her relatives, religious advisers, and other persons of standing, who, in turn, should be given every facility to meet the medical attendants if they so wish.

Organs from Cadavers

A. **Consent**
   Consent should normally be given in the following manner:

1. The deceased should provide recorded positive consent in his or her lifetime.
2. Failing to obtain consent from the donor who should be known not to have expressed opposition, consent from the next-of-kin should be sought.
3. Tissues may not be removed if there is a reason to believe that an inquest requires a post-mortem examination.
4. Immunological studies might be necessary during terminal illness of the prospective donor. Therefore, not only convenient, but also desirable to obtain the necessary consent before death has taken place.

B. Determination of Moment of Death

1. An individual who has sustained either (1) irreversible cessation of circulatory and respiratory functions or (2) irreversible cessation of all functions of the entire brain, including the brainstem. A determination of death must be made in accordance with accepted medical standards; this determination would be based as well on clinical judgment.
2. Pronouncement of death should be undertaken by two fully qualified practitioners, each independent of the team undertaking the transplant operation; at least one of the two practitioners must have been fully qualified for five years or more.

C. Corneal Grafting

In the case of removal of the cornea for grafting, the urgency is not similar to internal organs.

General Duties of the Doctor

Each medical act must be directed towards the absolute benefit of the patient, medically necessary and justifiable, carried out with the patient's approval or the approval of his guardian if he is a minor or unconscious[4].

Holding an Office

The doctor occupying a certain position is prohibited from using this position, whether it is administrative, political or social, for professional ends aimed at increasing the number of his patients. In addition, he/she is prohibited from using his post to obtain financial gain from his patients or receiving a fee for his services.

Advertising, Publicity and Commercial Enterprises

1. The doctor is prohibited from advertising, direct or indirect in various means, writing on signs, cards or labeling medical prescriptions or using a title which he did not receive legally.
2. The doctor is prohibited from resorting to means that may disgrace the medical profession, especially concerning fraud and claiming the discovery of new methods of diagnosis or treatment that are not scientifically proven.
3. The doctor is prohibited from writing in newspapers, magazines and using any other means of publishing in a way that may be considered as a personal advertisement.
4. Practicing any act that is in conflict with the integrity of the profession or doing any of the following:

    a. Allowing his name to be used in promoting medical drugs and various forms of treatment.
    b. Lending his name to commercial enterprises in any way.

c. Requesting or accepting a gratuity or fee for the prescription of medicines or the use of specific equipments.
   d. Giving consultations in a commercial magazine or in any of its supplements, which are intended to promote the sale of drugs or equipments or to recommend their use, whether such consultation was free or for a fee or bonus.

5. The doctor should not associate himself with commerce in such a way as to let it influence, or appear to influence, his attitude towards the treatment of his patients.
6. The Ethical Committee of King Hamad University Hospital disapproves the direct association of a medical practitioner with any commercial enterprise engaged in the manufacture or sale of any substance which is claimed to be of value in the prevention or treatment of a disease. These substances are recommended to the public in such a fashion as to be calculated to encourage the practice of self-diagnosis and self-medication or of undisclosed nature or composition.
7. The general public's interest in medical knowledge, the dissemination of medical information through radio and television, and the press interview, all demand the exercise of utmost caution by the doctor, whose professional standards condemn self-advertisement and publicity.
8. The public has a legitimate interest in the advances made in the science and art of medicine; it is of advantage that medical information discreetly be presented to the public through the media, for the particular purpose of "health education".
9. Great caution is necessary in public discussions on theories and treatment of disease owing to the misleading interpretation that may be put on these by an uninformed public. Sensational presentation should be avoided at all cost. The discussion of controversial medical matters, particularly about treatment, is more appropriate to medical journals or professional societies.

10. The use of advertising columns of the lay press to publicize the professional activities of individual medical practitioners, even in the absence of a name, is unethical.
11. Advertising the profession, in general, would certainly destroy those traditions of dignity and self-respect, which have helped to give the medical profession its high status. KHUH, therefore, draws attention to the danger of these objectionable methods and stresses the need for every member of the profession to offer a firm resistance to them.
12. The relationship of doctors with members of other medical professions must be marked by cooperation, respect and consideration of the benefits of all and such relationship should avoid causing any financial or moral harm and should avoid any course of action, which is not for the benefit of the patient or the profession. Any misunderstanding which arises in such a relationship must be raised to the Ethical Committee of KHUH.
13. The doctor may not have an interest in any pharmaceutical establishment, except holding ordinary shares in such a company. In addition, he may not receive a salary, commission or grant.

Doctor's Practice

The sharing of premises with members of allied professions, including professions supplementary to medicine, should be encouraged, but any infringement of free choice by the patient should be discouraged.

1. The doctor should organize a record for patients in which he/she registers the diagnosis, method, nature of treatment and observations.
2. Prescriptions must be very clearly written and fully worded with no ambiguity or vagueness and must contain a clear explanation of the method of administration.

3. Prescription forms may contain information as permitted by KHUH. Prescription forms must state the name and age of the patient as well as the date and must be signed by the doctor. However, in certain special cases, the name and age of the patient may be omitted.
4. The doctor is free to provide his services without charging a fee whenever his conscience compels him to do so. It is customarily recognized that the doctor would treat his relatives, friends, dependents, medical students, subordinates and assistants free of charge. However, the receipt of fees from some of those is not considered a violation of ethics.
5. The advertising of a specific time for free treatment is permitted; the doctor has the right to perform his duty without charging a fee for human reasons.
6. The period of treatment may not be preconditioned except in the case of pregnancy, surgery, physiotherapy and some exceptional cases related to surgery after obtaining the approval of KHUH.
7. The doctor is prohibited from sharing his fee with any of his colleagues except with whom he shares the treatment of a case.
8. Selling free medical samples whether to patients, other persons or establishments is forbidden.
9. A patient's life should not be ended, even if his affliction is terminal or how painful his affliction is or because the patient has become a burden to his family or those close to him.
10. The rules of this code apply equally to every doctor registered with KHUH and any violation of these rules exposes the violator to disciplinary action by the Ethical Committee in accordance with the established rules and regulations.

Sterilization

If the doctor is satisfied that an operation for sterilization is in the interest of the health of the patient and that the patient has given valid consent and understands the consequences of the operation; in the opinion of KHUH, there is no ethical reason why the operation should not be performed.

Considerations before Female Sterilization Procedure[5]

Female sterilization means obtaining permanent contraception by occluding the Fallopian tubes in women.

Informed Consent is Required

The following should be emphasized to the patient:

- Failure rate.
- Sterilization is an irreversible procedure.
- A woman must avoid sexual intercourse or use effective contraception until the menstrual period following the operation.
- Young females, especially below 25 years or those without children are more likely to regret.
- Couples with fewer than two children are more likely to regret.
- Relationship stability and break down.
- Tubal occlusion should be performed after an appropriate interval following pregnancy.
- Tubal occlusion postpartum or following an abortion has an increased regret and failure rate.

Vasectomy and Female Sterilization

- Vasectomy is a less invasive surgical procedure.
- Vasectomy is usually performed under local anesthesia.
- Consider manhood or womanhood in the Arab world before performing the sterilization procedure.

Alternatives to Sterilization

- Consider combined oral contraception (COC).
- Male condoms and caps but their reliability are poor.
- Coils-copper intrauterine contraceptive devices (IUCDs) can be used at any age.

Failure Rate of Female Sterilization

The failure rate is approximately 1:200, and there is an increased risk of ectopic pregnancy.

Complications of Female Sterilization

- Converting to an open procedure.
- Ectopic pregnancy.
- After the age of 30, female sterilization is associated with an increased rate of hysterectomy.

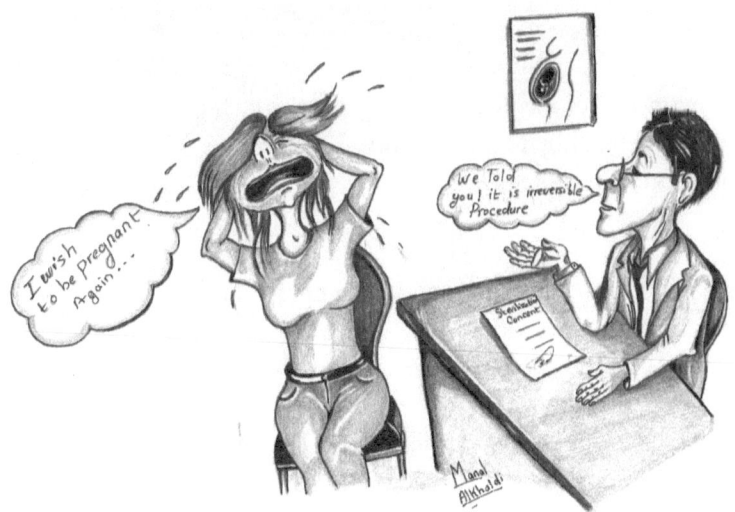

Duties of a Doctor towards Patients

"Medical responsibility towards the patient involves a commitment to caring, but there can be no undertaking to heal."

The doctor must, upon undertaking the treatment of any patient, do his utmost to provide dedicated care and compassion to all patients equally.

The doctor must uphold the following medical traditions[6]:

1. The freedom of the patient to choose the doctor.
2. The freedom of the doctor in prescribing, taking into consideration the financial condition of the patient.
3. Except in critical cases, the doctor has the right to refuse to give treatment for professional or personal reasons.
4. The doctor may discontinue treatment of his patient provided that:

    a. Such discontinuation does not harm the patient.
    b. All information necessary for the discontinuation of the treatment is provided.

The practice of medicine may require the giving of documents or reports defined by law. Each document of this kind must bear the signature of the doctor.

When preparing medical reports, the doctor must:

1. Abide by professional confidentiality except in cases defined by law.
2. Provide the reasons for writing the report.
3. Be objective and accurate and must exercise extreme caution.
4. Ensure that information contained in the report serve the required purpose.

5. Distinguish between information obtained as a result of his observation and diagnosis and information given by the patient or any other person. If he records the diagnosis of another doctor, he must write the name and address of the doctor in the report.
6. Clearly record the date of diagnosis, the date it was made and the signature and address of the doctor giving the report.
7. Make sure that it contains only medical information.
8. Keep in mind that giving a false medical report is unethical, and the doctor is liable to be prosecuted.

Suspected Death

In cases suspected to be criminal in nature, the doctor must inform KHUH legal authority who has the right to inform the legal authority in Bahrain to initiate post-mortem examination.

In criminal cases which end in death, the attending physician must refuse to give a death certificate and must inform the appropriate authorities.

Accidental deaths occurring in private clinics become the professional responsibility of the doctor, especially those occurring after minor surgeries, such as injections, operation on upper respiratory tract, anal operation, catheterization and antral washout. In such cases, the doctor is prohibited from giving death certificates and must immediately inform KHUH authority and the family of the deceased.

When it is not possible to give proper medical care, the doctor must, whatever his specialty is, give first aid to the patient whose life is in danger, unless there is some force compelling him not to.

If the doctor is requested urgently to treat a paralyzed minor or unconscious patient and could not promptly obtain the legal consent, then he must give the necessary treatment without any other consideration.

It is preferable not to hide the seriousness of the illness from the patient whenever possible. If concealed from the patient, the guardian must be advised of the seriousness of the illness.

The doctor must inform KHUH authority when he treats a patient contracting an infectious or contagious disease, such as HIV, Hepatitis, Tuberculosis, etc, in accordance with the laws.

The doctor is prohibited from performing an abortion by any method unless the continuance of the pregnancy constitutes a danger to the life of the pregnant woman or if deformity may result; in such circumstances, the following conditions must be met:

1. Abortion is performed by a specialist with the concurrence of another doctor.
2. The written report must be issued to determine the necessity of the abortion prior to performing the operation.
3. Four copies or more, as needed of the report must be issued and signed by the doctors, patient and spouse or guardian. The doctor and the family each have to keep a copy.
4. If the pregnant woman refuses to undergo the operation notwithstanding the doctor's explanation of the seriousness of her pregnancy, then he must comply with her wishes.

Professional Confidentiality

Professional confidentiality includes what the doctor learned of his patient's health and social conditions and what he may see, hear or understand from his patient as a result of his professional contact.

The doctor may not reveal without the consent of patient the information obtained during his professional relationship with the patient except if required by law.

Professional secrets may be revealed for the following reasons:

1. To the patient because the information concerns his illness or future.
2. To the guardian if the information concerns a minor or patient who is unconscious.
3. To the family of the patient if it is known that revealing this information would have a positive effect on the treatment.
4. If he is requested by the judicial authorities or in forensic cases.
5. For scientific purposes and medical research, without mentioning names or showing a defined picture.
6. The doctor may, during the performance of his medical duty, refer to previous medical conditions of the patient if he receives written request from judicial authorities allowing him to do so.

Other third parties who frequently seek information from a doctor are employers who request the medical condition of absent or sick employees, insurance companies requiring details about the history of life insurance or deceased policyholders and solicitors engaging in threatened or actual legal proceedings. In all such cases, the doctor should make it a rule to refuse to give any information in the absence of the consent of the patient or the nearest competent relative.

The Right of Your Colleagues

The relationship between doctors must be based on mutual respect and confidence which would facilitate ways of cooperation to serve patients and preserve the status of the profession[7,8].

The doctors must avoid anything that might harm their professional relationships and must endeavor to resolve their difference in an amicable manner, and if that proves impossible, the matter must be submitted to KHUH Ethical Committee.

A doctor is prohibited from publicly criticizing any of his fellow doctors or spreading rumors, which harm personality or have a harmful effect on professional practice. It is a sound professional practice to defend a falsely accused doctor.

A doctor is not allowed to attract other patients directly or indirectly and must not condone others doing this on his behalf.

A doctor has the right to receive any patient in his clinic without any commitment to the patient's previous physician.

A doctor must suggest medical consultation if the conditions of treatment require so, and must undertake the consultation if the patient or his family requests it. In both cases, the attending physician must recommend consultation with the doctor he sees most appropriate, taking into consideration the wishes of the patient.

A doctor is not allowed to manage a colleague's clinic temporarily for more than one month except after obtaining the approval of KHUH.

A doctor may not be represented temporarily for supervision and treatment of his patients except by a doctor registered with KHUH.

In cases where the patient is treated at KHUH, no other doctor may contact this patient concerning his treatment without the consent of the attending physician.

Ethical Machinery of KHUH

Disputes between Doctors

One of the most important functions of KHUH is to advise and assist employed physicians on ethical problems.

From time to time, doctors working together in a practice or in the same locality find themselves at variance with one another. Therefore, it is important that disputes should be immediately and amicably resolved within KHUH and whenever possible.

Disputes between a Doctor and Lay Person

The protection of individual medical practitioners against hostile attacks by members of the lay public or the press is one of the functions of KHUH where a lawyer could be provided.

Medical Protection

KHUH is obliged to provide lawyer protection for physicians practicing in the hospital.

The lawyer should be provided in all circumstances where there is a dispute on a medical matter.

All potential medico-legal cases should be reported to the Ethical Committee to take the necessary steps for the defense of the physician.

The Disciplinary Committee

The Disciplinary Committee consists of fourteen members. Twelve of them are consultants representing the different disciplines in the hospital. The remaining two members are non-professionals chosen by the twelve Disciplinary Committee members.

Infamous Conducts

The following conducts might lead to disciplinary action by KHUH:

1. Termination of pregnancy if done in circumstances which contravene the law in Bahrain.
2. Adultery or other improper conduct or association with a patient or a member of the patient's family.
3. Neglecting his professional duties to the patient.
4. Abuse of alcohol: A doctor might face a disciplinary action because of repeated convictions for drunkenness. It is customary to send a warning letter after the first conviction; a second conviction might lead to disciplinary action.
5. Abuse of dangerous drugs: disciplinary action might be initiated if a doctor breaches dangerous drugs regulations, or of some other offenses committed to gratify a doctor's addiction or a doctor convicted driving under the influence of a drug.
6. Untrue or misleading certificate and other professional documents: doctors are expected by KHUH to be extremely careful in issuing such documents. Any doctor who gives, in his professional capacity, any certificate or document containing statements which he knows or ought to know to be untrue, misleading or otherwise improper, may face a disciplinary action by KHUH Disciplinary Committee.
7. Covering up for or assisting an unqualified person to practice medicine.

8. Canvassing for the purpose of obtaining patients, whether it is done directly or through an agent.
9. Advertising: the professional offense of advertising may arise from the publication in any form or manner, commanding or drawing attention to the professional scale, knowledge, service or qualification.
10. Improper Financial Transaction:

    a. Accepting fees from a public patient;
    b. Receiving money which he is not entitled to;
    c. Commercializing of a secret remedy, improperly prescribing drugs or appliances in which a doctor has financial interest and arrangement for fees splitting.

11. The use of religion, nationality, race, party politics or social standing in the grounds of the hospital or allowing such things to intervene between the sacred duty of the physician and the patient.

KHUH Research Center

Criteria for Accepting Research Proposals in KHUH

1. The research should be conducted by health professionals in Bahrain.
2. The research should address common diseases or health care priorities in Bahrain.
3. The research should aim to increase our understanding of common diseases, their etiology, diagnostic or therapeutic interventions.
4. Applicant should submit a structured research proposal.
5. The research proposal should be scientifically sound and ethically acceptable.
6. The research should have been approved by the scientific and ethical committee at the investigator's institution.
7. The research proposals would be peer-reviewed to identify the high-quality research projects for funding.
8. The maximum amount of funding for any single research would be BD 4,000.

Research Proposal Format

The premise of the study

The title of the project: The title should be comprehensive, covering the main study objective(s) and study area.

Background: Literature review of previous studies on the subject (3-4 references only); justification of the study by stating the problem and its public health importance.

1. **Statement of the problem**
2. **Significance of the problem**
3. **Objectives of the study:**

   - **General Objective:** The aim of the study and goal that you need to achieve.
   - **Specific objective:** Detail of general objective.

Method: The method by which the study objectives could be best achieved.

- **Setting:** The area or setting where the study would be conducted.
- **Study subjects:** Inclusion and exclusion criteria for the study subjects.
- **Design:** Prospective, retrospective, analytic experimental: randomized clinical trials and non-randomized clinical trials. Analytic non-experimental: cohort, case-cohort, case control and cross-sectional, descriptive: a community survey, etc.
- **Sample size:** Mention the input criteria for sample size estimation. That might need the expertise of an epidemiologist.

- ➤ **Sampling technique:** Mention the sampling technique that would be used to obtain a representative sample of your target population. That might need the expertise of an epidemiologist.
- ➤ **The timeframe of the study:** The time needed to perform the study.

Data collection methods, instruments used and measurements: Describe the instruments to be used for data collection, such as questionnaire, observation recording form, etc.

Data management and analysis plan: Describe the overall plan and tests used for data analysis and the statistical package used.

Implications of the study results to population health and health system policy in KHUH and Bahrain: Expected results and potential contribution of the project to the decision making related to health care and policy in Bahrain.

References: Mention at least ten recent articles relevant to the study.

Ethical Consideration:

1. **Informed consent form:** If needed, please attach extra documents.
2. **Other funding agency:** Specify if your study is funded by another funding agency.

Preliminary Research Report: Should be submitted to the research committee after 3-6 months of research approval.

Final Research Report: The final report should be submitted in the form of a scientific article for publication.

Promotion of consultants and junior medical staff would be linked to study publication. In the case of junior medical staff, yearly publication is a precondition to be promoted to higher rank in the hierarchy of the medical ladder.

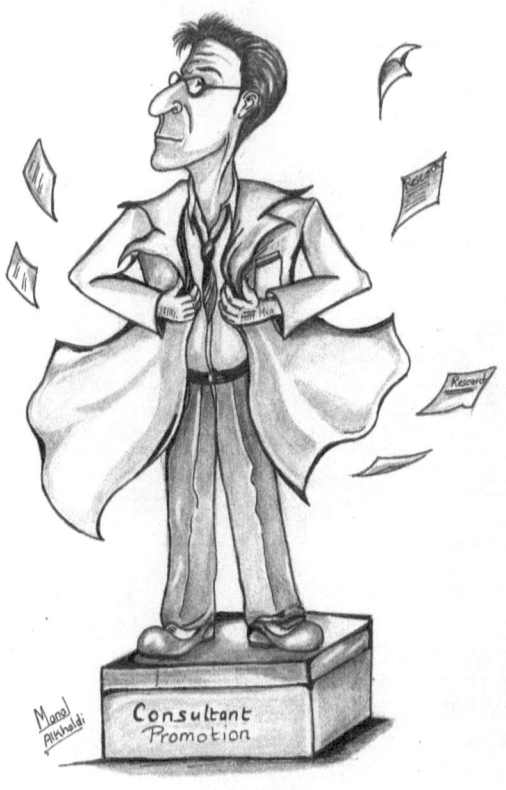

Research Proposal Application Form		
1. Title of the Study:		
2. Name of the Principal Investigator and Institutional Affiliation:		
Full name		
Occupation		
Place of Work		
Postal address:		
Telephone (office): Fax: Telephone (mobile): Email:		
3. Name and Signature of Other Investigators:		
1. Full name:		Email:
Tel(mobile):		Signature:
2. Full name:		Email:
Tel(mobile):		Signature:
3. Full name:		Email:
Tel(mobile):		Signature:
4. Full name:		Email:
Tel(mobile):		Signature:
Principal Investigator Signature:		
Official Use only **Scientific approval** ☐ Yes ☐ No **Ethical approval** ☐ Yes ☐ No		
Date of Receipt:		ID number:
Research Area:		
Referee 1: Referee 2: Committee Approval: ☐ Yes ☐ No Date:		
Budget requested from other sources: ☐ Yes ☐ No If yes, what is the source? Amount in BD:		

If you wish your research to be funded by KHUH, please include the following form.

Budget Breakdown	Amount in BD
1. Manpower	
Total manpower	
2. Services	
a. Laboratory	
b. Radiology	
c. Others (please specify)	
Total services	
3. Supplies and Equipment	
Total supplies	
4. Others	
Patients Cost	
Training	
Others (please, specify and justify)	
Total other	
GRAND TOTAL	
Investigators will receive 50% of the fund initially and the remaining 50% after submitting a progress report and completing data collection.	

Research & Ethics Committee Evaluation Form

Title: "_____"

Please complete and **sign** the checklist after reading the research proposal. Write your comments (if any) on the attached **comments form**.

STUDY DESIGN	Yes	No	N/A	Comments
TITLE				
Appropriate?				
Title is comprehensive and covers the main study objective(s)				
BACKGROUND & INTRODUCTION				
Appropriate?				
Significance of the problem is mentioned				
Is the aim clear?				
Statement of the problem is clear				
Appropriate length with references				
REFERENCES				
Citing of 10 references				
Conformity to *Vancouver* style				
Up-to-date (within the last 5 years)				
Relevant to the study				
METHOD				
Adequately described				
Study design is mentioned				
Sample size is done				
Eligibility and exclusion criteria of the study subjects are clear				
The instruments to be used for data collection is described				
Data management and analysis plan is/are described				
OVERALL RECOMMENDATION				
Clinical importance				
Satisfactory overall design				
English & writing style				
Informed consent (enclosed)				
Ethical consideration				
Potential contribution of the project to the health care in Bahrain is identified				

Priority of the Study   ❶ High   ☐ Acceptable without modification
                        ❷ Medium   ☐ Acceptable with modification
                        ❸ Low   ☐ Not acceptable

If not acceptable, please give a brief explanation on the back of this form

Date:
Name & Signature:
Research Committee Member

Variations of Informed Consent
Choose and modify as appropriate

Human Informed Consent Form-I

Instructions to the Researcher(s): An informed consent/assent/permission form should be developed in consultation with the adult sponsor, designated supervisor or qualified scientist[9].

This form is used to provide information to the research participant (or parent/guardian) and to document written informed consent, minor assent and/or parental permission.

- When written documentation is required, the researcher keeps the original signed form.
- Students may use this sample form or may copy ALL elements of it into a new document.

If the form is serving to document parental permission, a copy of any survey or questionnaire must be attached.

Researcher/s: _____
Title of Project: _____

I am asking your voluntary participation in my research project. Please read the following information about the project. If you would like to participate, please sign in the appropriate box below.

Purpose of the project: _____
If you participate, you would be asked to: _____
Time required for participation: _____
Potential risks of study: _____
Benefits: _____
How confidentiality would be maintained: _____

If you have any questions about this study, feel free to contact:

Researcher/Sponsor: _____ Phone/email: _____

Voluntary Participation:

Participation in this study is completely voluntary. If you decide not to participate, there would not be any negative consequences. Please be aware that if you decide to participate, you may stop participating at any time and decide not to answer any specific question.

By signing this form, I am attesting that I have read and understood the information above and I freely give my consent/assent for myself or my child to participate.

Adult Informed Consent/Minor Assent

Date Reviewed & Signed: _____

Printed Name of Research Participant: _____

Signature: _____

Parental/Guardian Permission: _____

Date Reviewed & Signed: _____

Parent/Guardian Printed Name:_____

Signature: _____

Genetic Sample Informed Consent-II

RESEARCH SUBJECT INFORMED CONSENT FORM

Project Information	
Project Title:	Project Number:
Site IRB Number:	Sponsor:
Principal Investigator:	Organization:
Location:	Phone:
Other Investigators:	Organization:
Location:	Phone:

1. PURPOSE OF THIS RESEARCH STUDY

➢ Include 3-5 sentences written in non-technical language, "You are being asked to participate in a research study designed to..."

2. PROCEDURES

➢ Describe procedures: "You would be asked to...".
➢ Identify any procedures that are experimental, investigational or non-therapeutic.
➢ Define expected duration of subject's participation.
➢ Indicate type and frequency of monitoring during and after the study.

3. POSSIBLE RISKS OR DISCOMFORT

➢ Describe known or possible risks. If unknown, state so.

- Indicate if there are special risks to women of childbearing age; if relevant, state that the study may involve risks that are currently unforeseeable to developing fetus.
- If subject's participation will continue over time, state: "any new information developed during the study that may affect your willingness to continue participation would be communicated to you."
- If applicable, state that a particular treatment or procedure may involve risks that are currently unforeseeable to the subject, embryo or fetus.

4. OWNERSHIP AND DOCUMENTATION OF SPECIMENS

- Describe ownership, use, disposal and documentation (identification) procedures for specimens or samples taken for study purposes.

5. POSSIBLE BENEFITS

- Describe any benefits to the subject that may be reasonably expected. If the research is not of direct benefit to the participant, explain possible benefits to others.

6. FINANCIAL CONSIDERATIONS

- Explain any financial compensation involved or state: "There is no financial compensation for your participation in this research."
- Describe any additional costs to the subject that might result from participation in this study.

7. AVAILABLE TREATMENT ALTERNATIVES

- If the procedure involves an experimental treatment, indicate whether other non-experimental (conventional) treatments are available and compare the relative risks (if known) of each.

8. AVAILABLE MEDICAL TREATMENT FOR ADVERSE EXPERIENCES

- ➤ "This study involves (minimal risk/greater than minimal risk)", if greater than minimal risk is involved, provide the subject with the following information.
- ➤ If you are injured as a direct result of taking part in this research study, emergency medical care would be provided by [name] medical staff or by transporting you to your personal doctor or medical center.

9. CONFIDENTIALITY

- ➤ Describe the extent to which confidentiality of records identifying the subject would be maintained. In addition, list steps to protect the confidentiality, such as codes for identifying data.

10. TERMINATION OF RESEARCH STUDY

You are free to choose whether or not to participate in this study. There would be no penalty or loss of benefits to which you are otherwise entitled if you choose not to participate. You would be provided with any significant new findings developed during this study that may relate to or influence your willingness to continue. In the event you decide to discontinue your participation in the study, these are the potential consequences that may result: (list)

- ➤ Please notify (name, contact details, etc.) of your decision or follow this procedure (describe), so that your participation could be orderly terminated.

In addition, your participation in the study may be terminated by the investigator without your consent under the following circumstances: Please describe them.

11. AVAILABLE SOURCES OF INFORMATION

- Any further questions you may have about this study would be answered by the Principal Investigator:

  Name:_____
  Phone Number: _____

- Any questions you may have about your rights as a research subject would be answered by:

  Name:_____
  Phone Number: _____

- In case of a research-related emergency, call:

  Day Emergency Number: _____
  Night Emergency Number: _____

12. AUTHORIZATION

I have read and understood this consent form, and I volunteer to participate in this research study. I understand that I would receive a copy of this form. I understand that my consent does not take away any legal rights in the case of negligence or other legal fault of anyone involved in this study. I further understand that nothing in this consent form is intended to replace any applicable laws.

- Participant Name (Printed or Typed): _____
- Date:_____
- Participant Signature:_____
- Date:_____
- Principal Investigator Signature:_____
- Date:_____
- Signature of Person Obtaining Consent:_____
- Date: _____

Informed Assent-III-Minor

An Informed Assent Form does <u>not</u> replace a consent form signed by parents or guardians. The assent is an addition to the consent and signals the child's willing cooperation in the study.

[Informed Assent Form for _____]

Name the group of individuals for whom this assent is written. Because research for a single project is often carried out on some different groups of individuals, such as children with malaria, children without malaria and/or students; it is important that you identify which particular group the assent is for.

(This informed assent form is for children between the ages of 12-16 who attend clinic X and who were invited to participate in research Y.)

[Name of Principal Investigator]

[Name of Organization]

[Name of Sponsor]

[Name of Project and Version]

This Informed Assent Form has two parts:

- ➢ **Information Sheet (gives you information about the study)**
- ➢ **Certificate of Assent (this is where you sign if you agree to participate)**

You would be given a copy of the full Informed Assent Form.

Part I: Information Sheet

Introduction

This is a brief introduction to ensure the child knows who you are and that this is a research study. Give your name, say what you do and clearly, state that you are doing research. Inform the child that you have spoken to their parents and that parental consent is also necessary. Let them know that they could speak to anyone they choose about the research before they make up their mind.

Objective: Why are you doing this research?
Explain the objective of the research in clear, simple terms:_____

Choice of participants: Why are you asking me?_____
Children, like adults, like to know why they are being invited to be in the research. It is important to address any fears they may have about why they were chosen.

Participation is voluntary: Do I have to do this?
State clearly and in child-friendly language that the choice to participate is theirs. If there is a possibility that their decision not to participate might be over-ridden by parental consent, this should be stated clearly and simply.

I have confirmed with the child/children and they understand that participation is voluntary:_____(initials)

Information on the Trial Drug [Name of Drug]: What is this drug and what do you know about it?

<u>Include the following section only if the protocol is for a clinical trial:</u>

1. Give the phase of the trial and explain what it means. Explain to the participant why you are comparing or testing the drugs.

2. Provide as much appropriate and understandable information about the drug, such as its manufacturer or location of manufacture and the reason for its development.
3. Explain the known experience with this drug.
4. Explain comprehensively all the known side effects/toxicity of this drug, as well as the adverse effects of all the other medicines that are being used in the trial.

Procedures: What is going to happen to me?
Explain the procedures and any medical terminology in simple language. Focus on what is expected of the child. Describe which part of the research is experimental.

I have confirmed with the child/children and they understand the procedures: _____(initials)

Risks: Is this bad or dangerous for me?
Explain any risks using simple, clear language.

Discomforts: Will it hurt?
If there would be any possibility of discomforts, state these clearly and simply. State that they should tell you and/or their parents if they are sick or are experiencing any discomfort or pain. Address some of the child's worries, for example, missing school or extra expense to parents.

I have confirmed with the child/children and they understand the possible risks and discomforts:_____(initials)

Benefits: Is there anything good that would happen to me?
Describe any benefits to the child.

I have confirmed with the child/children and they understand the benefits: _____ (initials)

Reimbursements: Do I get anything for being in the research?
Mention any reimbursements or forms of appreciation that would be provided. Any gifts given to children should be small enough, not as an inducement or reason for participating. WHO does not encourage incentives beyond reimbursements for expenses incurred, as a result of participation in the research. These expenses may include travel expenses and reimbursement for time lost. The amount should be determined within the host country context.

Confidentiality: Is everybody going to know about this?
Explain what confidentiality means in simple terms. State any limits to confidentiality. Indicate what their parents would or would not be told.

Compensation: What happens if I get hurt?
Describe to the ability of the child to understand and explain that parents have been given more information.

Sharing the Findings: Will you tell me the results?
Describe to the ability of the child to understand that the research findings would be shared in a timely fashion; however, confidential information will remain confidential. If you have a plan and a timeline for the sharing of information, include the details. Furthermore, tell the child that the research would be shared more broadly, such as in a book, journal, conferences, etc.

Right to Refuse or Withdraw: Can I choose not to be in the research? Can I change my mind?
You may re-emphasize that participation is voluntary.

Who to Contact: Who can I talk to or ask questions to?
List and give contact information for those people whom the child could contact easily (a local person who can be contacted). Tell the child that they could also talk to anyone they want to (their doctor, a family friend, a teacher).

If you choose to be part of this research, I would also give you a copy of this paper to keep for yourself. You could ask your parents to look after it if you want.

You can ask me any more questions about any part of the research study if you wish to. Do you have any questions?

PART 2: Certificate of Assent

This section could be written in the first person. It should include a few brief statements about the research and be followed by a statement similar to the one identified as 'suggested wording' below. If the child is illiterate but gives oral assent, a witness must sign instead. A researcher or the person going over the informed assent with the child must sign all assents.

I have read the information or had the information read to me; I have had my questions answered and I know that I can ask questions later if I have any.

I agree to take part in the research.

      OR

I do not wish to take part in the research and I have <u>not</u> signed the assent below.

_____ (initialed by child/minor)

<u>Only if child assents:</u>

Print name of the child: _____
Signature of the child: _____
Date: _____
      day/month/year

If illiterate:

A literate witness must sign (if possible, this person should be selected by the participant, not a parent and should have no connection to the research team). Participants who are illiterate should include their thumbprint as well.

I have witnessed the accurate reading of the assent form to the child and the individual has had the opportunity to ask questions. I confirm that the individual has given consent freely.

Print name of witness (not a parent): _____ **and thumb print of participant:**

Signature of witness: _____

Date: _____
       Day/month/year

I have accurately read or witnessed the accurate reading of the assent form to the potential participant and the individual has had the opportunity to ask questions. I confirm that the individual has given assent freely.

Print name of researcher:

_____

Signature of researcher:

_____

Date: _____
       Day/month/year

Statement by the researcher/person taking consent:

I have accurately read out the information sheet to the potential participant, and to the best of my ability, made sure that the child understands that the following would be done:

1.
2.
3.

I confirm that the child was given an opportunity to ask questions about the study and all the questions asked by him/her have been answered correctly and to the best of my ability. I confirm that the individual has not been coerced into giving consent and that the consent has been given freely and voluntarily.

A copy of this assent form has been provided to the participant.

Print Name of Researcher/person taking the assent: _____

Signature of Researcher/person taking the assent: _____

Date: _____
   Day/month/year

Copy provided to the participant _____ (initialed by researcher/assistant)

Parent/Guardian has signed an informed consent ____Yes. ____ No. ____ (initialed by researcher/assistant)

Informed Consent-IV-Parents

[Name of Principal Investigator]

[Informed Consent Form for _____]

Name the group of individuals for whom this consent is written. Because research for a single project is often carried out with some different groups of individuals, such as healthcare workers, patients and patients' parents; it is important that you identify which group this particular consent is for.

(This informed consent form is for the parents of children between 1 and 4 years of age who attend clinic Z and whom we are asking to participate in research X.)

Name of Principal Investigator:_____

Name of Organization:_____

Name of Sponsor:_____

Name of Proposal and Version:_____

This Informed Consent Form has two parts:

- Information Sheet (to share information about the study with you)
- Certificate of Consent for signatures if you approve the participation of your child.

You would be given a copy of the full Informed Consent Form.

PART I: Information Sheet

Introduction

Briefly, state who you are and explain that you are inviting them to have their child participate in research which you are performing. Inform them that they may talk to anyone they feel comfortable with about the research and that they could take the time to reflect on whether they want their child to participate or not. Assure the parent/s that if they do not understand some of the words or concepts that you would take the time to explain to them as you go along and that they could ask questions now or later.

Objective

Explain the problem/research question in lay terms which would clarify rather than confuse. Use local and simplified terms for a disease, such as the local name of the disease instead of malaria, mosquito instead of Anopheles, "mosquitoes help in spreading the disease" rather than "mosquitoes are the vectors". Avoid using terms like pathogenesis, indicators, determinants or equitable. There are guides on the internet to help you find substitutes for words which are overly scientific or are professional jargon.

Recognize that parents' feelings about involving their children in research could be complicated. The desire and feeling of responsibility to protect their child from risk or discomfort may exist alongside the hope that the study drug would benefit either their child or others. It is, therefore, important to provide clear and understandable explanations and to give parents time to reflect on whether they would consent to have their child participate.

Type of Research Intervention

Briefly, state the intervention if you have not already done so. This would be expanded upon in the procedures section.

Participant Selection

Clearly, state why their child was chosen to participate in this study. Parents may wonder why their child has been chosen for a study and may be fearful, confused or concerned. Include a brief statement on why children, rather than adults, are being studied.

Voluntary Participation

Indicate clearly that they could choose to have their child participate or not. State, <u>if it is applicable</u>, that they would still receive all the services they usually do if they decide not to participate. This could be repeated and expanded upon later in the form as well. It is important to state clearly at the beginning of the form that participation is voluntary so that the other information could be heard in this context.

<u>Include the following section only **IF** the protocol is for a clinical trial:</u>

Information on the Trial Drug [Name of Drug]

1. Give the phase of the trial and explain what it means. Explain to the parent why you are comparing or testing the drugs.
2. Provide as much information as is appropriate and understandable about the drug such as its manufacturer or location of manufacture and the reason for its development.
3. Explain the known experience with this drug.

4. Explain comprehensively all the known side effects/toxicity of this drug, as well as the adverse effects of all the other medicines that are being used in the trial.

Procedures and Protocol

It is important that the parents know what to expect and what is expected from them and their child. Describe or explain the exact procedures that would be followed on a step-by-step basis, the tests that would be done and the drugs that would be given. It is also important to explain from the outset what some of the most unfamiliar procedures involve, such as placebo, randomization, biopsy, etc. Describe very clearly which procedure is routine and which is experimental or research. Explain that the parent may stay with the child during the procedures. If the researchers are to have access to the child's medical records, this should be stated.

In this template, this section has been divided into two: first, an explanation of unfamiliar procedures and second, a description of the process.

A. **Unfamiliar Procedures**
   If the protocol is for a clinical trial:

   1. Involving randomization or blinding, the participants should be told what that means and what chance they have of getting which drug, such as one in four chances of getting the test drug. A very minimal statement is provided to give you an example. You may need to be more explicit about what is exactly involved.
   2. Involving a placebo, it is important to ensure that the participants understand what is meant by a placebo. An example for a placebo is given.
   3. May necessitate a rescue medicine, information must be provided about the rescue medicine or treatment, such as

what it is and the criterion for its use. For example, in pain trials, if the test drug does not control pain, then intravenous morphine may be used as a rescue medicine.

B. **Description of the Process**
Describe the process on a step-by-step basis.

In case of clinical research:

Explain that there are standards/guidelines that must be followed. If a biopsy would be taken, explain whether it would be under local anesthesia, sedation or general anesthesia, and what sort of symptoms and side effects the participant should expect under each category.

For any clinical study (if relevant):

If blood samples are to be taken, explain how many times and how much in a language that the person might understand.

If the tissues/blood samples or any other human biological material would be stored for a duration longer than the research purpose, or is likely to be used for a purpose other than mentioned in the research proposal, provide information about this and obtain consent specifically for such storage and use in addition to consent for participation in the study.

If not, explicitly mention that the biological samples obtained during this research procedure would be used only for this research and would be destroyed after ___ years, when the research is completed.

Duration

Include a statement about the time commitments of the research for the participant and the parent including both the duration of the research and follow-up, if relevant.

Side Effects

Parents should be informed if there are any known or anticipated side effects and what would happen in the event of a side effect or an unexpected event.

Risks

A risk could be thought of as being the possibility that harm may occur. Explain and describe any such possible or anticipated risks. Provide enough information about the risks that the parent could make an informed decision. Describe the level of care that would be available if harm does occur, who would provide it and who would pay for it.

Discomforts

Explain and describe the type and source of any anticipated discomforts that are in addition to the side effects and risks discussed above.

Benefits

Benefits may be divided into benefits to the individual, benefits to the community in which the individual resides and benefits to society as a whole as a result of finding an answer to the research question. Mention only those activities that would be beneficial and not those to which they are entitled regardless of participation.

Reimbursements

State clearly what you would provide the participants with for their participation. WHO does not encourage incentives beyond reimbursements for expenses incurred as a result of participation in research. The expenses may include travel expenses and reimbursement for time lost. The amount should be determined within the host country context.

Confidentiality

Explain how the research team would maintain the confidentiality of data, especially the information about the participant, which would otherwise be known only to the physician but would now be available to the entire research team. Because something out of the ordinary is being done through research, any individual taking part in the research is likely to be more easily identified by members of the community and is more likely to be stigmatized.

Sharing of the Results

Your plan for sharing the information with the participants and their parents should be provided.

If you have a plan and a timeline for the sharing of information, include the details. Also, inform the parent that the research findings would be shared more broadly, for example, through publications and conferences.

Right to Refuse or Withdraw

Reconfirm that participation is voluntary and includes the right to withdraw. Tailor this section well to ensure that it fits into the group for whom you are seeking consent. The example used here is for a parent of an infant at a clinic.

Alternatives to Participating

Include this section only if the study involves administration of investigational drugs or use of new therapeutic procedures. It is important to explain and describe the <u>established</u> standard treatment.

Who to Contact

Provide the name and contact information of someone who is involved, informed and accessible (a local person who could be contacted). State that the proposal has been approved and how.

PART II: Certificate of Consent

Certificate of Consent

This section should be written in the first person and have a statement similar to the one shown below. If the participant is illiterate but gives oral consent, a witness must sign. A researcher or the person going over the informed consent must sign each consent. The certificate of consent should avoid statements that have "I understand…." phrases. The understanding should perhaps be better tested through targeted questions during the reading of the information sheet (some examples of questions are given above), or through the questions being asked at the end of the reading of the information sheet, if the potential participant is reading the information sheet him/herself.

"I have been invited to have my child participate in research of a new malaria vaccine".

I have read the previous information, or it has been read to me. I have had the opportunity to ask questions about it and any question that I have asked had been answered to my satisfaction. I consent voluntarily for my child to participate in this study.

Print Name of Participant: _____
Print Name of Parent or Guardian: _____
Signature of Parent or Guardian: _____
Date: _____
        Day/month/year

If Illiterate

A literate witness must sign (if possible, this person should be selected by the participant and should have no connection to the research team). Participants who are illiterate should include their thumbprint as well.

I have witnessed the accurate reading of the consent form to the parent of the potential participant, and the individual has had the opportunity to ask questions. I confirm that the individual has given consent freely.

Print Name of Witness: _____AND
Thumb Print of Parent:

Signature of Witness: _____
Date: _____
        Day/month/year

Statement by the researcher/person taking consent:

I have accurately read out the information sheet to the parent of the potential participant, and to the best of my ability made sure that the person understands that the following would be done:

1.
2.
3.

I confirm that the parent was given an opportunity to ask questions about the study, and all the questions asked by the parent have been answered correctly and to the best of my ability. I confirm that the individual has not been coerced into giving consent and the consent has been given freely and voluntarily.

A copy of this has been provided to the participant.

Print Name of Researcher/person taking the consent: _____

Signature of Researcher/person taking the consent: _____

Date: _____
       Day/month/year

An Informed Assent Form would _____ OR would not _____ be completed.

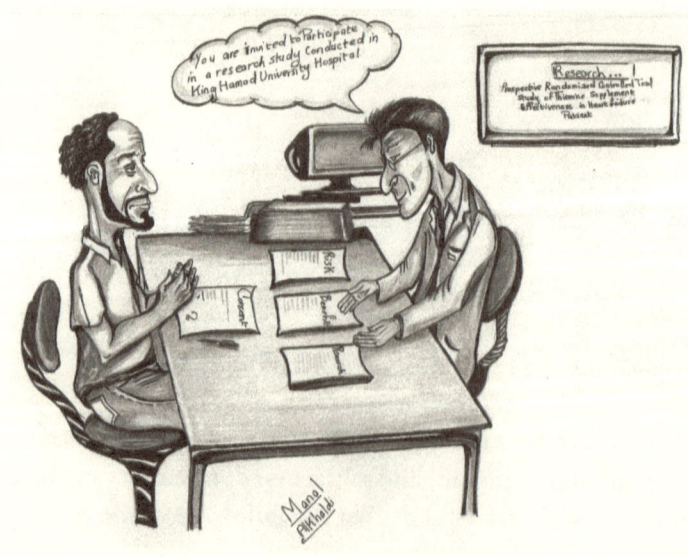

ETHICS AND THE LAW

Abdulla Alsowaidi

This chapter shall discuss ethics and in particular medical ethics and how it interrelates with the law. The objective of this chapter is to review briefly the difference between ethics and the law in general, as discussed in part I. The author shall evaluate two main ethical topics while making reference to Bahrain law and highlight the gaps in the current legislation. Finally, the writer shall briefly explain the process being followed for malpractice and medical negligence claims in Bahrain.

Part I: Ethics and the Law

Ethics are perceived by many to be doing what society accepts, or following the law or doing what feels to be right[1]. However, such perception is not entirely true as societies might not be in consensus on certain ethical matters, such as abortion; the law might deviate from ethical morality at certain times or in certain countries, and ethical values should not be perceived subjectively as one's perception differs from others[1]. Andrea and Velasquez defined ethics as standards that are objective, universal, consistent and based on good reasons, which describes what a human ought to do in a matter of right and wrong[2].

However, they also added that such ethical standards need to be constantly studied and reviewed about well-founded and reasonable grounds as time passes and new matters arise[2].

On the other hand, the law is defined as "the system of rules which a particular country or community recognizes as regulating the actions of its members and which may be enforced by the imposition of penalties"[3]. Thus, the law is regulated by the governing body in a country; it is applied to all citizens/residents of the country and it is enforced by imposing penalties on those who contravene it. While laws traditionally embody ethical principles, not all ethical standards are incorporated in the legal system and not all legislations and laws are based on ethical standards. Therefore, there is always a gap between laws and ethics as illustrated in figure 1.

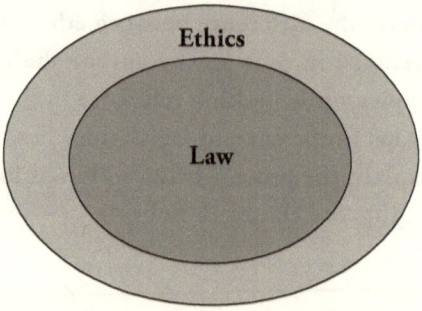

Figure 1: The Gap between Law and Ethics

This gap differs from one country to another; it expands and contracts from time to time, depending on the development and evolvement speed of both laws and ethics. While ethics cover a wider spectrum and evolve and develop at a faster pace, the law evolves at a much slower pace due to the lengthy process of changing regulations in most countries.

In light of such gap between the law and ethics, various professional associations, such as medical, legal and engineering associations and communities, have developed their code of ethics which codify the ethical principles that their members shall adhere to in their practice.

Such code of ethics is important due to the nature of the profession's practice and the fiduciary duty created between the profession's member and his/her subjects[4]. However, ethical codes are not legally binding by themselves, and therefore, laws are required to be enacted to create legal enforceability of such ethical principles.

The medical code of ethics is the most established and worldly recognized due to its importance. The Hippocratic Oath of the Fifth Century BCE is an oath taken by physicians, which is considered the oldest code of ethics and the patriarch of Western Medicine. Furthermore, Thomas Percival (1740–1804) published "Medical Ethics" in 1803, in which he defined the ethics to be followed by medical physicians. Such ethical principles became the basis for the first American Medical Association (AMA) in their first meeting in 1857. The AMA code of ethics consists of nine principles of medical ethics and various opinions on matters regarding physician's practice. However, such code of medical ethics is not law; nevertheless, practicing physicians must honor such principles.

AMA ethical principles became the basis for a code of ethics in various countries around the world. In Bahrain, there is no established and defined code of ethics by law; however, various Bahrain legislations have encompassed ethical principles. Nonetheless, the regulating authorities in Bahrain have adopted a code of medical ethics in 2007 which covers a wide range of ethical principles and has listed them under fourteen different sections[5]. The Bahraini code of ethics shall be discussed along with the relevant legislations in the following sections.

Part II: Bahrain Law

In this section, the author has selected two important ethical matters to be discussed. Under such discussion, the author shall make reference to the Bahraini legislations, Bahrain code of ethics (BCE) as well as AMA code of ethics (AMACE) to compare and analyze each ethical topic. The Bahraini legislations relevant to this chapter are Medicine and Dentistry Practice (MDP) Act (1989), National Health Regulatory Authority (NHRA) Act (2009) and Bahrain Criminal Code (BCC) (1976). The topics covered under this section are the following:

ABORTION

Abortion is defined as the deliberate termination of a human pregnancy, which leads to the death of the fetus[3]. BCE Articles 32 and 65 state that a physician is prohibited from conducting, recommending, assisting or initiating an abortion procedure unless the aim behind such procedure is the preservation of the mother's life from severe harm and only after consulting a specialized physician as per the MDP regulations. The regulations as per the MDP Article 19 states: "a doctor has no right to prescribe medicine (drugs) that leads to abortion or to perform an abortion procedure unless continuation of the pregnancy will threaten the life of the pregnant woman". Article 19 stated four conditions for abortion to be performed:

1. Three registered consultants must agree to and approve the abortion.
2. Abortion must be performed by a doctor specializing in obstetrics and gynecology.
3. Abortion must be performed in a public hospital or authorized private hospital.
4. The pregnant woman legal guardian consent to the abortion.

AMACE states under Opinion 2.01 that a physician is not prohibited from performing an abortion in accordance with good medical practice and under circumstances that do not violate the law[6].

Considering the above-mentioned references, the Bahraini legislations consider abortion illegal unless the conditions stated are met. AMACE states that abortion is not prohibited to be performed provided that such procedure does not violate the law. It can be inferred from the above that all medical code of ethics are primarily consistent in the abortion matter, and the Bahraini legislations cover most of the aspects related to the abortion procedure. However, the Bahraini legislations are only allowing abortion in the case of pregnancy causing a life-threatening condition to the pregnant woman, whereas other countries extend the approval for an abortion for pregnancies resulting from rape, incest, fetus abnormalities or threat to the physical health of the woman[7].

In addition, there are some aspects in which the Bahraini legislations have not been covered:

- **Counseling before the abortion procedure:** such step is followed in various countries to ensure that the woman is aware of all the risks and matters involved in undergoing an abortion, such as the link between abortion and breast cancer, the ability of a fetus to feel pain and psychological consequences for undergoing such procedure[5].
- **Waiting period:** imposing mandatory waiting period between the consultation at the clinic and the abortion procedure. That allows the pregnant woman to have sufficient time to consider the procedure[7].

In summary, the matter of abortion is substantially covered by Bahraini legislations and the BCE. Nonetheless, the legislations require updates to cover other aspects which are found in other countries.

Palliative and End of Life Care

The World Health Organization (WHO) defined Palliative Care as an approach that improves the quality of life of patients and their families facing the problem associated with life-threatening illness[8]. Another definition by National Cancer Institute (NCI) is that palliative care is given to improve the quality of life of patients who have a serious life-threatening disease, such as cancer[9]. The term "Palliative Care" and "End of Life Care" shall be used interchangeably for the purpose of this section.

The objective of the "End of Life Care" is to focus on the comfort of patients rather than treatment. The National Council for Palliative Care (NCPC) summarized the objectives of palliative care as follows[10]:

- ➤ Affirm life and regard dying as a normal process
- ➤ Provide relief from pain and other distressing symptoms
- ➤ Integrate the psychological and spiritual aspects of patient care
- ➤ Offer a support system to help patients live as actively as possible until death
- ➤ Offer a support system to help the family cope during the patient's illness and in their own bereavement

BCE Article 31 states that a physician shall not waste a life or induce the death of a person even for compassionate reasons. However, Article 33 states that patients suffering from irreversible conditions and are at the end of life, a physician shall do his/her best for the end of patient's life with dignity, comfort and respect.

In contrast, the Bahraini legislations have not made any specific reference to the end of life care. The legislations focused on the physician's duty to treat, Article 24 of MDP states that "a doctor must not refuse to treat or aid an injured patient unless the medical case is out of the doctor's field of specialization or for valid reasons." The BCC states "any doctor who refuses to treat a patient will be subject to a prison sentence of six months to ten years depending on the severity of the medical case."

AMACE have a more liberal approach regarding the end of life care as it states "Physicians are not ethically obligated to deliver care that, in their best professional judgment, will not have a reasonable chance of benefiting their patients. Patients should not be given treatments simply because they demand them. Denial of treatment should be justified by reliance on openly stated ethical principles and acceptable standards of care."

In consideration of those mentioned above, it is clear that the Bahraini legislations have not adequately dealt with the end of life care, and it creates confusion and some concerns for physicians as it does not provide a clear rule in such critical matter. The MDP legislation imposed an obligation to treat all patients and gave a broad exemption if valid reasons exist. However, the BCC creates a contradiction as it does not accommodate for such exemption and impose punishment for refusal to treat. However, the BCE gives a better understanding of the current stand, though it does not have any legal standing, and therefore, there is still a risk of prosecutions for doctors refusing to treat end of life patients.

Nonetheless, this gap could be filled by reference to Islamic jurisprudence as a source of legislations in Bahrain. There are some Islamic rulings in which it gave clear guidance on the obligations of physicians towards the end of life patients. In particular, the decision of the Islamic Fiqh Council (1996) states that it is permissible to remove life support machines if:

- ➢ The heart and lungs cease to work and the physicians agreed that this cessation is irreversible.
- ➢ The brain ceases to function completely, and specialized physicians agreed that this cessation is irreversible, and the brain started to deteriorate.

In addition, the Permanent Committee of Scholarly Research and Ifta (1988) gave similar ruling by stating that if it is evident that a patient's brain is irreversibly damaged, as agreed by three specialized and qualified physicians, then life support may be removed and relatives of the patient's views shall not be taken into consideration as they are not specialized in the field.

Furthermore, for patients with irreversible illness, such as stage IV cancer with very poor prognosis (often six months or less), the

Permanent Committee of Scholarly Research and Ifta (1988) states that once three specialized and qualified physicians agree that a patient falls under such description of irreversible condition, then it is permissible to categorize such patients as "do not resuscitate".

In conclusion, the legislations in Bahrain have to cater for the end of life care as this matter is not properly addressed and there is no unified process in hospitals to be followed towards the end of life patients. This might cause physicians to be reluctant to stop treating patients and shifting them to "do not resuscitate" status because of the fear of possible prosecution. In addition, this will create a further burden on hospitals resources to continue support end of life patients[6].

Part III: Legal Claims for Malpractice and Medical Negligence

In this section, the author shall discuss the current process of legal claims in relations to malpractice of medical negligence. The MDP Article 27 states that a physician is not responsible for curing a condition in a patient if the doctor has provided all the necessary treatment and took all the required steps in diagnosing and treating the patient.

However, a doctor is liable in the following situations under Article 27:

> - If a doctor made an error that caused harm to the patient due to lack of knowledge in some technical or practical aspects which a doctor is supposed to know.
> - If a patient was harmed due to the doctor's negligence or not providing proper patient care.
> - If a doctor conducted scientific research or study unauthorized by NHRA, which may cause harm to the patients.

If a physician contravenes any of the obligations under BCE or MDP, which constitutes a negligence or malpractice, then a claim process shall be initiated as shown in figure 2.

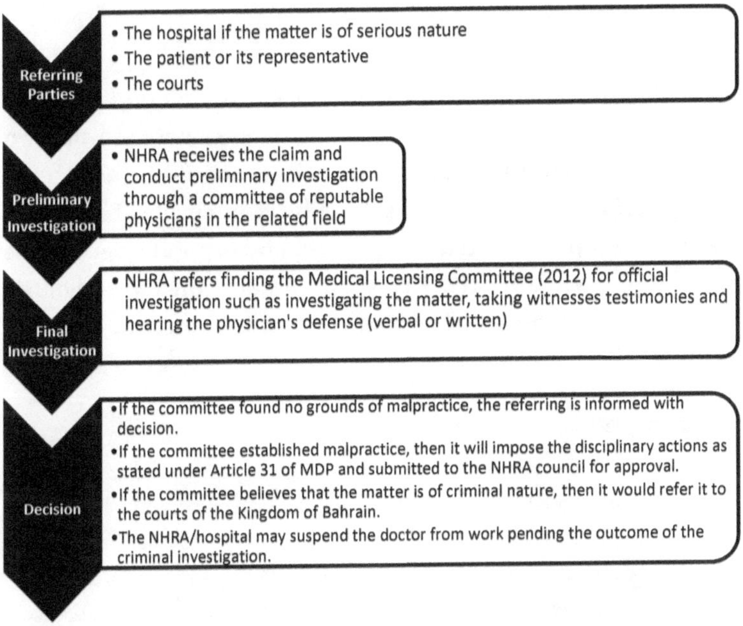

Referring Parties
- The hospital if the matter is of serious nature
- The patient or its representative
- The courts

Preliminary Investigation
- NHRA receives the claim and conduct preliminary investigation through a committee of reputable physicians in the related field

Final Investigation
- NHRA refers finding the Medical Licensing Committee (2012) for official investigation such as investigating the matter, taking witnesses testimonies and hearing the physician's defense (verbal or written)

Decision
- If the committee found no grounds of malpractice, the referring is informed with decision.
- If the committee established malpractice, then it will impose the disciplinary actions as stated under Article 31 of MDP and submitted to the NHRA council for approval.
- If the committee believes that the matter is of criminal nature, then it would refer it to the courts of the Kingdom of Bahrain.
- The NHRA/hospital may suspend the doctor from work pending the outcome of the criminal investigation.

Figure 2: Malpractice and Medical Negligence Claims Process

The MDP Article 31 states that the disciplinary actions in which NHRA is authorized to take against a physician regarding malpractice or medical negligence as shown in figure 2 are the following:

- ➢ Written warning
- ➢ Suspension from practice up to one year
- ➢ Disbarring and terminating the doctor's practice license

The claims process provide adequate steps towards reaching a decision. However, there must be a proper education for healthcare workers as well as patients of such process. That would help to channel claims properly and reduce the current trend of initiating claims in the courts.

CONCLUSION

This chapter provides a brief insight of the relation between ethics and the law by discussing the difference between the two and how it is vital that ethical principles should be enshrined in legislations for such principles to be enforceable. The law in Bahrain requires continuous updates to incorporate legislations which addressed ethical matters such as abortion and end of life care to support the healthcare workers in the country.

REFERENCES

1. Corrigan RH, Farrell ME. Ethics: A University Guide. Progressive Frontiers Pubs; 2010, USA, 361.
2. Markkulla Center for Applied Ethics. What is Ethics? http://www.scu.edu/ethics/practicing/decision/whatisethics.html Accessed January 2016.
3. Oxford Dictionary of English. 3rd ed. Oxford University Press. http://www.oxfordreference.com/view/10.1093/acref/9780199571123.001.0001/a cref-9780199571123 Accessed January 2016.
4. Frank A. Riddick, Jr. The Code of Medical Ethics of the American Medical Association. Ochsner J. 2003 Spring; 5(2): 6–10.
5. Ministry of Health. Bahrain Code of Medical Ethics. 2007.
6. AMA Council on Ethical and Judicial Affairs. Code of Medical Ethics of the American Medical Association. https://www.ama-assn.org/about-us/code-medical-ethics Accessed January 2016.
7. Guttmacher Institute. An Overview of Abortion Laws. https://www.guttmacher.org/state-policy/explore/overview-abortion-laws Accessed January 2016.
8. World Health Organization. WHO Definition of Palliative Care. http://www.who.int/cancer/palliative/definition/en Accessed January 2016.
9. Palliative Care in Cancer. National Cancer Institute. http://www.cancer.gov/about-cancer/advanced-cancer/care-choices/palliative-care-fact-sheet Accessed January 2016.
10. Patients and Carers |NCPC. http://www.ncpc.org.uk/patients-carers Accessed January 2016.

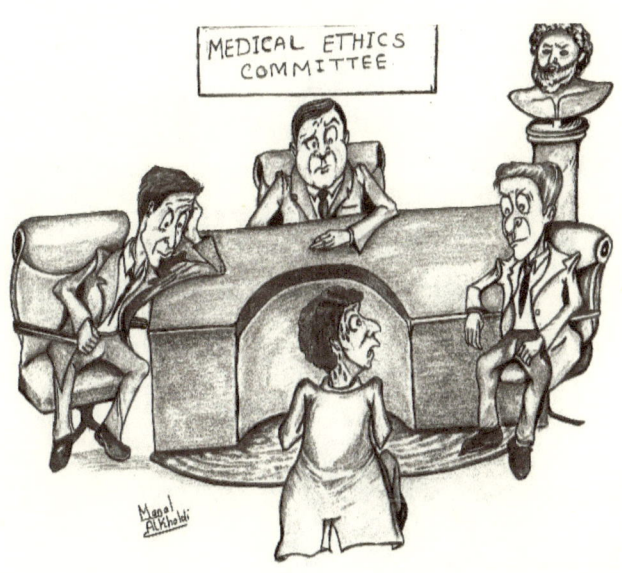

CONSENT

Martin T. Corbally

We live in an era where patients are rightfully entitled to participate in any and all decisions concerning physical examination, treatment, intervention or investigation. That imposes significant responsibility on the physician who must balance such advice based on the risk and benefit of the attendant and must present this information in a meaningful and understandable way. Consent must be obtained before commencing any treatment or investigation and inherently implies excellent communication and adherence to ethical principles. Consent and its expanded form "informed consent" are enshrined in national and international laws primarily to protect the patient but very important also the doctor.

While consent is vital in all research on human subjects, it is dealt with elsewhere in this book and needless to say that it is of equal and often of superior importance. While focusing on consent as it relates to practice, this chapter will deal with informed consent, the right to refuse treatment and consent in certain complex situations.

What Is Consent?

By definition, consent underlines a mutual agreement (from the Latin con "together" and Sentire "feel") to provide treatment (doctor) on the one hand and to receive or refuse it (patient) on the other. It is a principle that is rooted in the philosophical notion of autonomy and is a vital and indispensable component of clinical practice. All patients have the right to agree or refuse treatment, and it behooves the physician to respect that right at all times. This may sometimes appear at odds with the absolute duty of a physician to improve the health of patients when competent individuals refuse such treatment. However, as much as it is a doctor's duty to save lives and ease suffering and pain, it is equally so to abide by a patient's decision even when this may place the patient at risk. In reality, legal systems recognize the dilemma that a physician might face in this situation and have provided various mechanisms to protect the doctor with recourse to the courts when necessary.

However, autonomy, as a philosophical concept, is not always absolute and has limited (vide infra) utility when applied to minors and those of unsound mind or limited mental capacity. The family is recognized in law as the arbiter of responsibility and consent when dealing with minors, but the courts also recognize and respect the decisions and opinions of minors when this does not conflict with a preventable negative outcome. In practice, it is wise to include minors when explaining risk/benefit issues and seeking consent. In some cultures, this may also include the extended family.

Why Is Consent Necessary?

Consent is based on the philosophical notion of autonomy and essentially means that all human beings (patients) have the ability and right to rationalize their decisions and to refuse or accept treatment. Such freedom of choice does not infer a judgment or analysis of consequence, which could be difficult for doctors to accept knowingly that a refusal to accept a prescribed treatment may compromise outcome or survival. In essence, consent must be obtained for every intervention, and a doctor could be found guilty of assault if consent had not been properly acquired. Consent (vide infra) is implied when a patient presents for physical examination or consultation, and it is not normally necessary to obtain written consent for examination; it would be unwise of any physician to proceed without obtaining verbal consent to examine the patient. That takes on even greater significance in some cultures. However, when considering consent, we are mostly addressing consent for a procedure, interventional treatment and certain investigations.

The concept of consent and the absolute right to information about treatment has changed dramatically since Holmes in 1861; in "Currents and Counter-Currents in Medicine", he stated, "Your patient has no more right to all the truth than he has to all the medicine in your saddle bags"[1]. This has gradually been replaced by an awareness that physicians must obtain consent for all elective procedures and that the patient is entitled to make that choice. That concept was elegantly outlined in law in the case of Schlondorff versus Society of New York Hospital in 1914 in making an enlightened judgment which stated, "Every human being of adult years and sound mind has a right to determine what shall be done with his body, and a surgeon who performs an operation without the patient's consent commits an assault"[2]. Although various embellishments have been added and developed around this theme, it remains the core definition of consent in modern medical practice. Treating a patient without consent violates their rights and may result in a criminal charge against the doctor. Generally, consent need not be obtained in emergency situations where there is a clear risk to life or limb. Nevertheless, it is always best to have made an effort to secure such consent if time and situation allow.

How Should Consent Be Obtained?

In general, consent is either written or verbal; while most would agree that written consent is superior as it clearly underlines risk/benefit and provides a legal record, it is also acceptable to obtain verbal consent, such as telephone consent, when it is not possible to obtain it in writing. In this situation, it is prudent to have verbal consent witnessed and a written note made of the interaction.

For the most part, when we speak of consent, we consider two forms: expressed or implied. An example of the latter is when a patient attends a clinic and is aware that an examination is part of the normal process. There is no formal requirement to obtain anything in writing, as in this case, actions speak louder than words. However, caution must be exercised especially when intimate examination is required, and the physician would be well-advised to confirm consent for this examination but also sensible to have this examination performed in the presence of a chaperone.

Consent might also be implied, meaning that it is not necessary to obtain it, in emergency situations where there is a risk to life or limb or where the patient is unconscious or has altered comprehension as a result of injury. The courts would normally accept that the physician has acted in the best interest of the patient, but if possible, it is always best practice to attempt to obtain consent or at least inform the next of kin.

Implied consent should be used carefully during surgical procedures where the surgeon performs another procedure for which he has not obtained consent. It could and should only be relied on when the surgeon encounters an unanticipated condition that would pose a significant risk to the patient if not removed or dealt with. It is never appropriate to perform a surgical procedure because the surgeon happens to be there and it is a matter of convenience only. These concepts were developed in Mohr versus Williams in 1905, which in essence stated that the surgeon is justified to rely on implied consent when failure to deal with an unanticipated intraoperative finding would place the patient at subsequent serious risk.

In Mohr versus Williams, the surgeon obtained consent for surgery on one ear but noted intraoperatively that the other ear was the one in need of surgery[3]. Although he performed a successful surgery on the non-consented ear, he was nevertheless found to have committed an assault. That also underlines the principle in law that even though, the outcome was very positive; the patient could sue and win on a charge of assault.

Fortunately, doctors are rarely charged with criminal assault in matters where consent is challenged and are more likely to be found guilty of negligence. A charge of assault may still apply; however, if there has been deliberate misinformation given to the patient or in some way the patient has been deliberately misled. In other words, the principle of implied consent must never be used for the sole reason of convenience, but is reserved for situations of risk to life and limb.

Consent should be obtained by a doctor who understands the planned procedure, its risks and benefits and the consequences of refusal to accept this treatment. The ideal person would normally be the consultant or the surgeon performing the operation. In practice, that may not always be practical or feasible in most hospitals. To accommodate that, most systems allow for consent to be obtained by a nominated and competent deputy who is of sufficient experience to provide appropriate information on the procedure or intervention. Hospitals often overcome the deficiency by having team briefings to highlight any issues with consent; however, it is essential that any concern regarding procedural consent be addressed to the most senior physician.

Essential Components of Consent

The essential components of consent are the following:

1. Provide the patient with all the information that they need to make an informed decision about their medical treatment.
2. Answer all questions honestly and to the best of your ability.
3. If uncertain about the accuracy of any answer, refer to a colleague of superior experience, but never knowingly give the patient inaccurate information.

4. Communicate in a language that is non-medical and easy for the patient to understand.
5. Frequently check that the information is understood and retained.
6. Allow a reasonable period (days or weeks) for the patient to process and research the provided information.
7. If possible, provide information leaflets compiled in easy to understand language.
8. Respect the patient's right to reject or accept any treatment you recommend without consequence to the patient.
9. Always be prepared to recommend and facilitate a second opinion to a physician of the patient's choice.

Consent is properly viewed as a dynamic exchange of information between the provider (Doctor) and the patient. It is dynamic in that the patient has the right to enquire and/or question any and all aspects of the information being given. Similarly, the physician undertakes to provide all relevant information to the best of their ability, and if uncertain about any aspect, they must refer to a more experienced or senior colleague. Patients must fully participate in this process which describes the inherent risks (see below under informed consent) and the anticipated benefits. It is equally important that potential alternatives are described and in the presence of perceived uncertainty that the patient may always be entitled to avail of a second opinion. From a legal perspective, consent must be given or withheld voluntarily by an individual of legal capacity and must flow from an exchange of appropriate information.

Informed Consent

It is likely that every medical practitioner is aware of the need to discuss informed consent with every patient, but it is almost certainly the case that many are unclear as to what it means. Doctors are frequently unsure of how much or how little detail is required to fulfill the criteria of informed consent, and it seems that, at times, the courts themselves are uncertain where the appropriate balance lies. In general, the completeness of informed consent would be decided when compared against what a reasonable doctor would describe or conversely what a reasonable patient would expect to be told. There are clearly limitations to both definitions especially where the medical profession is judged to decide the basis of what is a reasonable doctor. Perhaps the most sensible way to define adequate informed consent is the one in which a patient would consider material to their decision to proceed with a procedure or not. If it could be shown that the information given to the patient was inadequate to the point where he/she would not have given consent if greater detail had been known, then informed consent may not have been complete. In Roger's versus Whittaker, the plaintiff argued that the consent would have been withheld had they been informed of the risk; however, rare contralateral blindness is in the non-operated eye[4].

In losing this case, it was clear that the doctor had a duty to inform the patient of a material risk of complete blindness, which occurred as a result of this very rare complication. There was no issue of incompetence; merely the duty to inform the patient who as a reasonable individual may well have decided that the risk to quality of life (total blindness) was too great to agree to this elective procedure.

Concerning risk, it is important that the person obtaining consent does so in a clear manner using a language the patient understands. A description of risk should include the side effects of the procedure, the potential for failure of the procedure and the consequences of not undergoing the procedure. Debate continues as to the extent of informed consent necessary and whether each and every side effect should be disclosed as the list could be extensive and be the cause of significant anxiety. There is no procedure without risk and some carry greater risk than others. As a general rule, the greater the material risk, the more obligated is the need to discuss it. In the absence of this discussion, the courts are likely to find favor with the doctor only if it is considered that a reasonable patient would have agreed even in the absence of this disclosure.

What Are the Special Circumstances?

On occasions, the doctor would be faced with challenges in obtaining informed consent. This includes:

> ➢ The patient does not want to know the details.
>
>> This is a rarely encountered situation, as today the majority of patients wish to be informed of their condition and its treatment. However, if a patient wishes to sign a consent, but does not wish to be informed, how should the doctor proceed? In this rare event, it is important that adequate time is given to the patient who may have adopted this approach out of anxiety. Detailed explanations may not be in the patient's interest if likely to cause undue mental distress or anxiety. However, it is advisable to seek help and assistance from a social worker or psychologist and to inform a senior consultant or high-level administrative officer of the problem especially when there is a valid concern that the information may be harmful to the patient. In all such cases, it is important to provide basic information and to document all aspects of the consent process, including that the patient did not wish to hear further detail.

If the Patient Is a Minor (Underage)

In a general sense, parents are regarded as the advocates of their children's rights and while children have, under European law, the right to liberty, bodily integrity and to communicate with others and follow their conscience, it is understood that most jurisdictions impose thresholds and circumstances where consent for children is directed by parents. The law could, at times, be confusing especially where the legal age of consent and that of adult autonomy are different (see Child Care Act 2001 and section 23 of the Non-Fatal Offenses against the Person Act 1997, Ireland)[5]. The distinction is further blurred where consent for medical or social treatment may be legally given in the absence of parental consent if the child has sufficient understanding of the implications of the treatment[6]. Clearly, there are cultural and jurisdictional differences that impact on how the law treats consent in minors and the reader would be best served to become familiar with what is relevant to their region.

Essentially, children are normally regarded as incapable of consenting to any treatment or refusing treatment where that refusal may have a serious and irreversible consequence. The age limit would vary from country to country but always has, at its core, the well-being of the child. In some situations, a parental belief may interfere with the rights of the child, such as refusal to allow blood transfusion in some religions, and the judiciary may be obliged to intervene, although this is uncommon. As summarized in Prince versus Massachusetts 1944, "Parents may be free to become martyrs themselves, but it does not follow that they are free in identical circumstances to make martyrs of their children before selves"[7].

In all cases involving consent for minors, it is important to include the minor in the consent process and to ensure significant understanding by the child. That is important when the child is in adolescence stage and has expectations to be treated as such.

Mental Capacity and Consent

In all cases, it is vital that the patient has a clear understanding of the planned treatment, its benefits, risks and alternatives. An individual's ability to understand, consent or refuse treatment must not be based on their appearance, underlying medical diagnosis, such as dementia, beliefs, ethnic background, language, age or religion. It is always based on the patient's ability to understand and retain the information given and the ability to use that understanding to make an informed choice. In some cases, a thorough assessment of the capacity is required if consent is being obtained for a major operation and may be less so for minor interventions, such as a new medication. Normally, doctors work on what is called a presumption of capacity and only when there is a suspicion that this is not so the case that alternative strategies are used. Patients who suffer from dementia may have a lucid interval, for that period they are considered as having full capacity. In general, capacity must be called into question when they are unable to understand the process offered, could not retain and question the discussion, or make choices that seem based on a misperception of reality. In this case, advice may be sought from those close to the patient while seeking advice from the Hospital's Ethics Committee. The decision to proceed may be assisted by the courts when time allows or deferred if the procedure is an elective and not vital to the patient's wellbeing.

CONCLUSION

Consent is an absolute requirement for any procedure or investigation and demands excellent communication between the patient and the practitioner. It demands a clear and straightforward explanation in terms which the patient understands. Failure to acquire consent may result in a charge of assault against the doctor because failure to obtain adequate consent may result in a charge of negligence. Information to the patient must be freely given and never withheld, and the patient's right to an explanation and second opinion always upheld. In essence, the doctor should not adopt a paternalistic view and be open and frank with the patient including detailing risks, benefits and potential for failure of the procedure. Consent is a dynamic process that involves the doctor and the patient with information unfolding as the patient's needs are met.

REFERENCES

1. Holmes OW. Currents and Counter-Currents in Medicine: With Other Addresses and Essays. In: Mills S, eds. Clinical Practice and the Law. 2nd edition. UK: Tottel Publishing, 2007: 73.
2. http://www.lawandbioethics.com/demo/Main/LegalResources/C5/Schloendorff.ht m Accessed July 2016.
3. http://www.lawandbioethics.com/demo/Main/LegalResources/C5/Mohr.htm Accessed July 2016.
4. Chalmers D, Schwartz R. Rogers V. Whitaker and Informed Consent in Australia: A Fair Dinkum Duty of Disclosure. Med Law Rev 1993; 1(2):139-59.
5. http://www.irishstatutebook.ie/1997/en/act/pub/0026/sec0023.html#sec23 Accessed July 2016.
6. http://www.hrcr.org/safrica/childrens_rights/Gillick_WestNorfolk.htm Accessed July 2016.
7. https://supreme.justia.com/cases/federal/us/321/158/case.html Accessed July 2016.

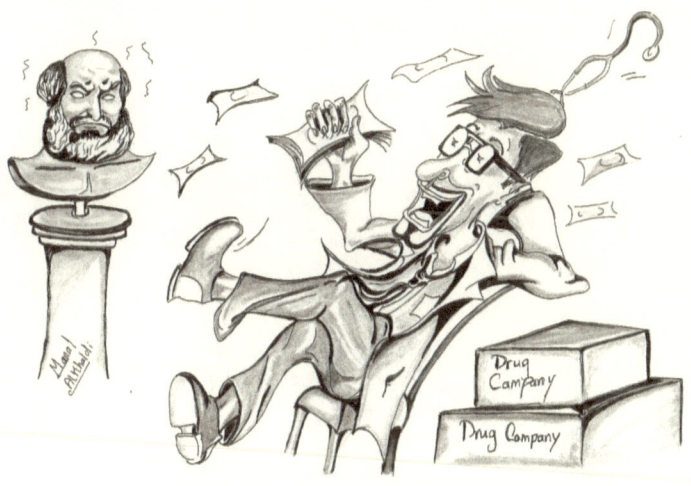

TEACHING ETHICS TO MEDICAL STUDENTS AND RESIDENTS: THE METHODS AND CHALLENGES OF PASSING MEDICAL ETHICS TO FUTURE PHYSICIANS

Dalal Alromaihi

Medicine has always been considered a moral profession. Good clinical practice should not be separated from professional and ethical behavior that depends on moral maturity[1].

The fundamental justification for teaching clinical medical ethics is based on its contribution to patients' care. Providing medical care goes far beyond the ability to diagnose and treat; good medical care provides the best care with equality while minimizing harm and taking into account the patients' needs and rights. In educating young physicians, the ethics of the decision-making process should be considered more than the ethics of the actual decision[2].

Medical ethics should be taught by competent teachers and those who could motivate the students and residents. Academic physicians are well-suited because they could teach ethics in the clinical setting. Physicians are responsible for identifying and resolving clinical and ethical problems. A physician with ethically appropriate professional attitudes and values would provide a role model to students and residents.

The Evolution of Medical Students' and Residents' Ethical Behavior

Medical students usually begin medical school as young idealists; however, many are challenged during medical education and clinical practice, which may lead to moral stunning or regression[3-8].

Evidence from a questionnaire revealed that there is limited moral maturity among medical students compared to their peers in other settings[7]. A survey of medical students also confirmed that the majority feel that their moral values are eroded during the clinical years[8]. In one survey, 74% of residents have directly observed mistreatment of patients[9].

Faced with ethical dilemmas or challenges, the students and residents might assume an attitude of apathy towards these challenges as they have been exposed to them repeatedly or a positive one, where maturity takes place. Students and residents who were observed to have adopted the attitude of apathy are no longer affected by the emotional aspect of such ethical challenges. In addition, when the clinical load increases and burnout ensues, apathy is an adaptive behavior noted in some residents and physicians as they progress in their clinical experience. Those who have adopted a positive attitude, on the other hand, reveal maturity. Applying what they have learned based on their previous experiences, the identification of ethical dilemmas and challenges becomes easier and the ability to respond to them professionally evolves into a second nature. Our responsibility as medical educators is to create an innovative learning environment and curriculum to motivate young physicians to embrace the latter attitude effectively and to continue with the same passion throughout their clinical careers.

Early Methods of Teaching Medical Ethics

Prior to 1970, medical ethics education occurred mainly through observation; these principles were transmitted from physicians to students in traditional apprenticeship model of medical education.

Only few medical schools taught medical ethics as separate formal courses. By 1989, the proportion of medical schools that had separately required courses had risen to 34%, such as in the United States[10]. Many of the pioneers of formal medical ethics education began their careers as teachers of moral philosophy or theology[11]. The model used back then was based on formal classroom sessions, and it was directed towards allowing the students to recognize, clarify, analyze and debate ethical issues.

Current Methods of Teaching Ethics

Certain teaching practices have become popular and mainstream, resulting in what we call the traditional model of medical ethics education. According to the traditional model, it is not the role of the ethics teacher to teach personal traits, such as courtesy, empathy and compassion. Rather, medical ethics education should augment the student's future clinical competence with the knowledge and cognitive skills necessary for ethical decision-making. Although traditionalists hope and expect that the intellectual tools gained in medical ethics courses would be put to sound practical use, the traditional model is essentially analytic, emphasizing the process of moral deliberation more than its conclusions.

The goals and methods of medical ethics education have grown progressively broader and more complex. The field's goals have begun to reach beyond identifying and analyzing ethical issues into the realm of influencing students' attitudes and behaviors. Its methods have expanded to incorporate an impressive range of new teaching techniques. The main current teaching methods are summarized herein.

Role Modeling

Role modeling method is usually used for teaching students and residents ethical behavior.

Students and residents identify most positively with mentors who are enthusiastic and those with outstanding clinical skills and teaching abilities[12-16]. Negative role models are identified as the faculty who are dissatisfied with their carriers and display poor interpersonal interactions with patients and others[17]. It is important in role modeling to include mutual learning goals and allowing the teacher to highlight behaviors that are being modeled along with accurate feedback on the modeled behaviors. It is important to foster positive role modeling among clinical faculty. This approach is supported by studies that students are more profoundly affected by role models than by formal coursework[18-19].

Formal Lectures and Workshops

Formal lectures are still frequently employed as a standard method of teaching ethics. A popular method is to combine large group presentations with small group discussions. While much of medical ethics education is still devoted to teaching conceptual knowledge and analytical skills, some curriculums teach specific behavioral skills as well. This development followed from the notion that even the best-intentioned students may not always be adept at translating theory into practice.

Humanism in Medicine Peer Support Groups

One approach is based heavily on humanistic qualities, and the concepts are derived from psychology and social sciences. This approach usually makes use of longitudinal peer support groups that encourage students to discuss the stress of becoming a doctor. It may also include other structured activities, such as role-playing sessions, meeting with faculty advisors or stress management training[20-23].

Role Playing Method

Role model playing method is where students watch each other in role-play of delivering bad news, obtaining consent and discussing "do not resuscitate" orders. Students are then asked to compare the observed techniques and discuss a list of practical suggestions.

Challenges of Teaching Ethics to Medical Students and Residents

The main challenge of addressing students' ethical development is the numerous ranges of influences on that development. One of the few areas of universal agreement concerning students' development is that medical training could make students and residents more cynical and insensitive. Our role as medical educators is to continue to enforce the highest standard of integrity.

Teaching ethics is a challenge when the institution is commercially driven or falls under the pressure of financial constraints where priority services may contradict the ethical concepts being taught. Another challenge is in busy practices where time is limited for a demonstration of ethical conducts, as clinicians are obliged to service a large number of patients and less time is allocated to reflect on ethical dilemmas identification and resolution.

As the strategies of performing medicine and evaluating physicians' performance in developed countries shift from quality to quantity with a focus on see more and do less, more strain is placed on ethical conduct and demonstration to medical students and residents.

Strategies to Enhance the Effectiveness of Teaching Ethics

There are some general principles in medical education to enhance the mentors' ability to teach students and help them retain and retrieve that knowledge and skills effectively and apply it when needed. The following methods highlight and strengthen our ability to teach ethics to medical students and residents.

Teaching Should Be Clinically-Based

Teaching the principles of ethics to medical students and residents is similar to teaching the concepts of diagnosis and therapy to be meaningful to their future medical practice. Teaching ethics must be clinically-based as it relates to their day-to-day work in the clinic, wards and research laboratories. Therefore, teaching should be clinically-oriented preferably case-based scenarios, where the real patient or clinical cases should serve as the teaching focus.

Teaching Should Be Continuously Reinforced during Their Training

Ethics teaching should be integrated during the years of medical students and residency training.

The best time to teach brain death and the vegetative state is during neuroanatomy and neurophysiology courses. Anatomy course offers a unique opportunity to deal with issues of death and respect for the dead body. The doctor-patient relationship, truth-telling, confidentiality and informed consent should be dealt with during history taking and physical diagnosis course[2].

Teaching Ethics Should Be Structured and Systematic

Clinical medical ethics teaching should include cognitive training in the fundamentals of ethics with a core set of lectures on important topic areas. To complement it, students and residents could be referred to a recommended text that is clinically oriented along with a bibliography of accessible articles and reference materials for further reading.

Clinicians Should Ultimately Serve as the Instructors

Clinicians should be the teachers and role models for the students. In evaluation forms of clinicians, with whom students and residents rotate, some questions should be added to evaluate their capabilities to serve as role models in ethical conduct and demonstration of professionalism. Feedback on their performance in such areas would have an impact in assigning more trainees with them or not.

Faculty Development Programs with Focus on Teaching Ethics

Such programs are needed to emphasize the role of moral education and the education of ethics. That should improve the ability of faculty to pass ethical principles to students and residents[23-25].

Emphasizing Interdisciplinary Collaboration

The interdisciplinary education underscores the need for physicians to value the perspective of people from varying backgrounds and set an example for subsequent inter-professional collaboration. One popular strategy is to have teams of clinicians and non-clinicians teach cooperatively.

Demonstrating Importance of Learning Ethics

It is important to emphasize to students and residents that learning ethics is as important as learning other components of the medical curriculum. That is demonstrated by featuring ethics teaching sessions prominently in the requirements and emphasizing on it throughout the curriculum rather than listing it lower in the priority of importance.

In conclusion, teaching ethics to medical students and residents is of utmost importance in providing excellence in medical care. There are several challenges to conducting such teaching, but with the availability of several teaching models and strategies, the influence of such challenges could be minimized. It is our responsibility as medical educators to foster an environment that supports teaching such concepts and continuously behave as role models for the upcoming stride of young physicians.

Dr. Dalal Alromaihi was awarded the Role Model Award for Medical Students from Wayne State University and the Award of Humanism in Medicine from the Arnold P. Gold-Gold Humanism Honor Society in 2009.

REFERENCES

1. Branch WT Jr. Supporting the Moral Development of Medical Students. J Gen Intern Med 2000; 15(7):503-8.
2. Siegler M. Lessons from 30 Years of Teaching Clinical Ethics. Virtual Mentor 2001; 3(10).
3. Branch W, Pels RJ, Lawrence RS, et al. Becoming a Doctor. Critical-Incident Reports from Third-Year Medical Students. N Engl J Med 1993; 329(15):1130-2.
4. Hupert N, Pels RJ, Branch WT Jr. Learning the Art of Doctoring: Use of Critical Incident Reports. Harvard Student BMJ 1995; 3:99-100.
5. Feudtner C, Christakis DA. Making the Rounds. The Ethical Development of Medical Students in the Context of Clinical Rotations. Hastings Cent Rep 1994; 24(1):6-12.
6. Christakis DA, Feudtner C. Ethics in a Short White Coat: The Ethical Dilemmas that Medical Students Confront. Acad Med 1993; 68(4):249-54.
7. Self DJ, Baldwin DWC Jr. Moral Reasoning in Medicine. In: Rest JR, Narváez D, eds. Moral Development in the Professions: Psychology and Applied Ethics. Hillsdale, NJ: Lawrence Elbaum Associates, 1994: 147-62.
8. Feudtner C, Christakis DA, Christakis NA. Do Clinical Clerks Suffer Ethical Erosion? Students' Perceptions of Their Ethical

Environment and Personal Development. Acad Med 1994; 69(8):670-9.
9. Baldwin DC Jr, Daugherty SR, Rowley BD. Unethical and Unprofessional Conduct Observed by Residents During their First Year of Training. Acad Med 1998; 73(11):1195-200.
10. Stemmler EJ. Teaching Medical Ethics: A Hard-Won Beachhead. Acad Med 1989; 64(12):704.
11. Jonsen AR. Medical Ethics Teaching Programs at the University of California, San Francisco, and the University of Washington. Acad Med 1989; 64(12):718-22.
12. Ambrozy DM, Irby DM, Bowen JL, et al. Role Models' Perceptions of Themselves and Their Influence on Students' Specialty Choices. Acad Med 1997; 72(12):1119-21.
13. Wright S. Examining What Residents Look For in Their Role Models. Acad Med 1996; 71(3):290-2.
14. Wright S, Wong A, Newill C. The Impact of Role Models on Medical Students. J Gen Intern Med 1997; 12(1):53-6.
15. Reuler JB, Nardone DA. Role Modeling in Medical Education. West J Med 1994; 160(4):335-7.
16. Wright SM, Kern DE, Kolodner K, et al. Attributes of Excellent Attending-Physician Role Models. N Engl J Med 1998; 339(27):1986-93.
17. Mutha S, Takayama JI, O'Neil EH. Insights into Medical Students' Career Choices Based on Third- and Fourth-Year Students' Focus-Group Discussions. Acad Med 1997; 72(7):635-40.
18. Pellegrino ED, Hart RJ Jr, Henderson SR, et al. Relevance and Utility of Courses in Medical Ethics. A Survey of Physicians' Perceptions. JAMA 1985; 253(1):49-53.
19. Sulmasy DP, Terry PB, Faden RR, et al. Long-Term Effects of Ethics Education on the Quality of Care for Patients Who Have Do-Not-Resuscitate Orders. J Gen Intern Med 1994; 9(11):622-6.
20. Self D. The Pedagogy of Two Different Approaches to Humanistic Medical Education: Cognitive Vs Affective. Theor Med 1988; 9:227-236.
21. Puckett AC Jr, Graham DG, Pounds LA, et al. The Duke University Program for Integrating Ethics and Human Values into Medical Education. Acad Med 1989; 64(5):231-5.

22. Kiser K. Students with a Heart. The Gold Humanism Honor Society Urges Medical Students to Doctor with their Hearts as Well as their Heads. Minn Med 2007; 90(8):16-7.
23. Wilkerson L, Irby DM. Strategies for Improving Teaching Practices: A Comprehensive Approach to Faculty Development. Acad Med 1998; 73(4):387-96.
24. Hundert EM, Hafferty F, Christakis D. Characteristics of the Informal Curriculum and Trainees' Ethical Choices. Acad Med 1996; 71(6):624-42.
25. Fox E, Arnold RM, Brody B. Medical Ethics Education: Past, Present, and Future. Acad Med 1995; 70(9):761-9.

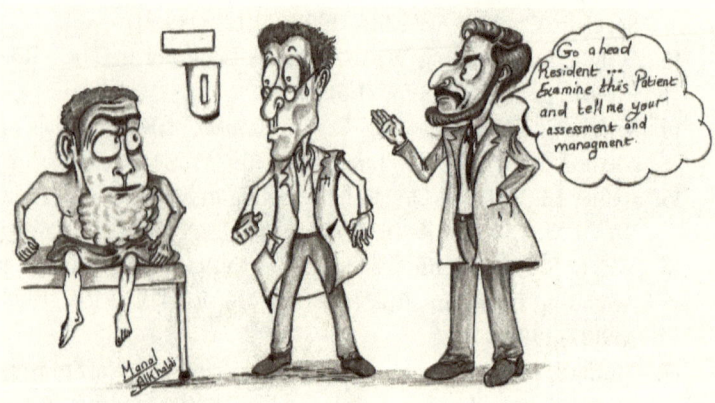

END-OF-LIFE CARE POLICY

Eamon Tierney, Hamdy Abozenah

Medical Terminology at the End of Life Care

The greatest challenge surrounding any discussion regarding end-of-life care is the lack of understanding of what "end-of-life care" means. Terms such as "end-of-life care", "do not resuscitate (DNR)", "allow natural death", "do not attempt resuscitation (DNAR)", "palliative care", "non-escalation of care", "terminal care" and even the word "euthanasia" are commonly grouped without full understanding of the exact meaning of the terms[1].

As physicians, we are obliged not only to understand the terms, but also to use them carefully, especially in front of families, whose understanding would usually be influenced mainly by the media. The use of the term "DNR" could have an explosive effect when mentioned to families, as they wrongly but frequently associate it with euthanasia, "pulling the plug" or simple abandonment of the patient. Some physicians themselves fail to understand the meaning of these terms, and could differ greatly in their interpretations. In a study from King Hamad University Hospital in Bahrain, physicians were asked anonymously to list their understanding of the term "DNR" regarding basic issues as pain relief, feeding, nursing care, antibiotics, etc. It was evident that there was a wide interpretation of what DNR meant and a small number of physicians' opinions were frightening. One physician understood DNR to mean that pain relief should be withheld from the patient[2].

The term DNR means "Do Not Resuscitate," but what is resuscitation? Resuscitation is frequently misinterpreted as the actions that are carried out after a cardiopulmonary arrest, such as intubation of the airway, administration of artificial breaths, chest compressions, etc. However, resuscitation means so much more than that. Resuscitation includes administration of fluids, feeding, oxygen and symptomatic relief - measures that are designed to sustain life as well as to restore it. The term "fluid resuscitation" is used for patients who are dehydrated, have been bleeding or who have suffered burns[3]. Therefore, if an end-of-life care patient is dehydrated, he would, of course, be resuscitated with fluids, although he would not be resuscitated using chest compressions and electric shocks.

Perhaps the term "end-of-life care" is more appropriate than "DNR" when a decision is made that further treatment of a patient is futile. End-of-life care means that all ordinary nursing and medical care would be given to a patient to ensure his comfort and to relieve any symptoms he may have. Therefore, the patient would be fed with appropriate calories, given full nursing care and physiotherapy, and administered medications that would render him more comfortable, such as analgesics, anti-emetics, laxatives and psychoactive medications to relieve anxiety or depression. However, the patient would not be given further treatment to cure the disease because it is beyond treatment.

End-of-Life Care for Cancer Patients

End-of-life care is applied and accepted in areas such as oncology. Most lay people are aware of cancer patients who received surgery, chemotherapy and radiotherapy, but at some point in their management, after they had developed secondary tumors in the lungs, liver, bones or brain, the treating physicians made a decision that further active treatment was futile; from then on, palliative care or relief of symptoms, would be carried out. Most people accept this as normal practice. Society has an understanding of cancer and accepts the ethical correctness of end-of-life care or palliative care in this area without difficulty.

The "Inoperable" Patient

Most people have also experienced a situation where a patient presents to a surgeon with a condition where, although the surgeon deems the patient in need of surgery, decides that the condition is "inoperable" because of the overall condition of the patient, the co-morbidities or the hopeless prognosis of the presenting condition. That means that the patient would not have his core condition dealt with, but would have symptoms relief. That is a classic application of end-of-life care and is a concept that is accepted by most people. An example of this might be a person with multiple co-morbidities presenting late with a superior mesenteric artery thrombosis. This condition leads to a large amount of dead bowel and is always incompatible with survival when it presents late. An operation is technically possible, in that one could open the patient's abdomen and remove the dead bowel; however, survival is impossible. The public accepts the concept of the "inoperable" patient, just as it accepts end-of-life care in a cancer patient. Occasionally, physicians see a problem in an end-of-life patient and feel that it could be technically treated by an operation or procedure. While this may be technically correct, they fail to see the overall picture of hopelessness, and they forget that the patient would need anesthesia, intensive care and major organ support, with a hopeless prognosis, which could cause undue suffering to the patient. These physicians are thinking more like technicians rather than discerning professionals.

End-of-Life Care in the Intensive Care Unit

There is a need to develop a plan of care in patients who are critically and irreversibly ill at an end-stage of illnesses other than cancer or an inoperable surgical problem. Usually, these patients are in an

Intensive Care Unit and have been receiving intensive management of their illness until a point is reached where the illness becomes irreversible and further treatment is futile.

A patient with end-stage respiratory failure in the ICU usually had a long history of severe respiratory illness and respiratory failure, and is now in the ICU with an acute exacerbation of the respiratory failure, and is on a ventilator. Attempts at weaning the patient off the ventilator have repeatedly failed. The patient would have developed further complications of his respiratory failure, such as overwhelming sepsis, cardiac failure and failure to respond to repeated antibiotic therapy and other therapies for respiratory care. At a point where the medical ICU team considers further treatment futile, the team should be allowed to continue ventilation, continue feeding via tube and continue administration of fluids and appropriate sedation to the patient; however, other measures, such as dialysis and cardiac support should not be undertaken.

Families find it more difficult to accept the concept of end-of-life care in this environment, perhaps because people nowadays have higher expectations that illnesses that cause ICU admission could be cured. These families would often have an acceptance of end-of-life care in cancer or inoperable patients. However, they would be unfamiliar with ICU scenarios. In some ways, it is hard to blame them. The most common cause of death in the ICU is sepsis; however, the public expects that infection could be successfully treated with antibiotics. It is difficult to persuade them that the common ICU pathogens nowadays could be resistant to many of the available antibiotics and that there is a lot more to the management of sepsis and septic shock than antibiotics.

The continued futile treatment of a dying patient in an ICU causes unnecessary discomfort to the patient, unnecessary distress to the family and professional discomfort and ethical difficulties for the medical team. Physicians should not be obliged to perform pointless procedures on patients whom they consider to have no hope of survival, and they should not engage in this behavior voluntarily. That goes against the basic medical ethical principle of *"Primum non nocere,"* but is frequently carried out because of fear that the family or hospital management would punish them if they do not continue treatment. There should be an acceptance of the concept of an illness reaching an "end point" beyond which, life might be artificially extended for a short period using extraordinary means, such as a ventilator or drug infusion. In such cases, purposeful lifespan is not extended. Physicians who recognize this stage of illness should institute end-of-life care. Continuation of futile care is unethical practice, even if the family wants it, as it is not in the patient's best interest. The challenge is to persuade the family of the correct course of action, rather than allow or expect the family to decide the medical treatment, which would be inappropriate.

A satisfactory term for care at the end-of-life in an ICU environment is "non-escalation" of care. Since the patient is already critically ill in the ICU, one could assume that the patient is attached to a ventilator, on multiple infusions of drugs and perhaps also having renal replacement therapy. It is clear that some of these treatments could not be stopped suddenly, as the immediate death of the patient would ensue. Patients on ventilators develop a dependence on ventilators; even the healthiest patients need to be weaned slowly from a ventilator. Sudden disconnection of a ventilator would usually cause death. Therefore, a system of end-of-life care that works well in the ICU is non-escalation – the level of artificial support of the patient would not be increased from the moment of the decision to institute end-of-life care; however, neither would it be reduced. This non-withdrawal and non-escalation of therapy would satisfy all ethical requirements.

Implementing an End-of-Life Care Decision

To implement end-of-life care is clearly a major decision and should always be carried out in accordance with a written hospital policy.

In 1974, the American Medical Association (AMA) made history by being the first medical organization to recommend that the decision not to resuscitate be documented formally in a patient's notes and that the instruction should be communicated to all physicians involved in the patient's care[4]. The first such policies to be published in medical journals were by the Massachusetts General Hospital and the Beth Israel Hospital, both in Boston in 1976[5].

The end-of-life care policy should be an open document available for all to see. Patients and their families should know where they could access it on a hospital website. There should be no element of secrecy or subterfuge about it. Damage has been done in the past to end-of-life care when patients or families were not informed that it had been implemented. As recently as May 2016, the issue of "secret" end-of-life care reached the media in the UK, and such incidents destroy the confidence of the public in the medical profession[6].

The end-of-life policy must be strictly adhered to. There are criteria regarding which types of patients might be considered for end-of-life care and these are outlined in the policy document. If a patient does not fall into one of the categories listed, he should not be considered for end-of-life care. In addition, the number of physicians making the decision and their ranks are key aspects of the policy. At King Hamad University Hospital, the policy states that two consultants must be involved in the decision and must write the decision in the patient's record. In practice, the entire team of ICU physicians, coming from different religious and cultural backgrounds, make the decision. When a plan of end-of-life care is first discussed in the ICU and when the agreement is obtained amongst the ICU team, the admitting consultant is approached and asked for an opinion. If the admitting consultant agrees, the end-of-life care plan would be written into the notes by an ICU consultant and by the admitting consultant. The ICU team never implements end-of-life care on its own and always seeks confirmation from other specialties.

Discussing End-of-Life Care with the Patient's Family

The question of whether the family should be involved when end-of-life care is instituted on a patient is a difficult one. The key answer is that the family should be kept informed of the patient's condition in the ICU daily before end-of-life care becomes an issue. Poor communication on the part of physicians is one of the biggest misdemeanors of modern medicine, and poor communication could also be a major problem in the ICU. If a family is communicated daily, a relationship of trust is established between the medical team and the family. However, the technique of talking to the family needs to be carefully thought out. The family must always be told the truth. It is good to give hope to a family, but wrong to give false hope. Patients and families need to be able to believe that physicians, more than any other professional, would always tell the truth. Physicians should never meet a patient or family alone or in a corridor. The meetings should always be formal in an office where privacy is assured, and at least two members of the ICU team should be present, as well as the nurse caring for the patient, if possible. Formal introductions should take place, as the family needs to know with whom they are talking, and clearly the physicians need to know that the person with whom they are speaking has the authority to receive patient information. At each meeting, the conversation should begin by asking the family how they feel the patient is doing that day. That gives the physicians an idea of the family's understanding of the gravity of the patient's condition. The physicians should then explain the current condition, outlining the gravity of the situation and the poor prognosis. Too much intricate medical detail should be avoided, as the family would not be able to put changes in numerical values into perspective. If the family is given clinical numbers, then when the creatinine falls from 200 to 199 the family would think that there has been an improvement. The key issues that determine the patient's outcome, should be explained in detail, but minor issues should not be emphasized. If a patient has suffered major brain damage following a vascular insult, detailed explanations of the ulcers in his digestive tract are unnecessary and confusing to the family. The conversation should concentrate on the issue that would impact most on the patient.

At the end of each daily meeting, questions from the family should be encouraged and answered honestly. It is acceptable to admit that one does not know the answer to a particular question. In the case of a dying patient, a standard question would be: "How much longer would my mother last?" Giving a definite answer to this is not only arrogant and foolish, but it also leads to a loss of credibility and trust when one is ultimately proven wrong. Attempts by a physician to be able to see into the future are doomed to failure. It is acceptable, however, to say something like "In my experience, in the ICU environment, patients such as your mother only last a few days, but every patient is different, and one never knows for sure." Similarly, when families ask whether they should call in family members living abroad, the criticality of the patient's condition should be re-emphasized, the prognosis should be provided according to previous experience, and the family could make the decision to call in members from abroad.

When the ICU team makes the decision that end-of-life care is appropriate and a non-escalation plan of management should be instituted, the family should be informed in a formal meeting. There are several reasons why the family itself could not make the decision of non-escalation. The physicians have the knowledge, training and experience in these matters. The first obligation on the part of the medical team is towards the patient, not towards the family; allowing the family to insist on continuing full treatment of the patient in a futile manner would be an abandonment of the rights and needs of the patient by the medical team.

A family would not be able to make such a decision of non-escalation easily. They do not have the medical knowledge required and would rarely be able to achieve unanimity on such a decision. If the decision were to fall on one member of the family, such as the patient's spouse or eldest child, the pressure on them to make an end-of-life decision would be unreasonable and unfair.

Frequently, a family member would cite religious objections to initiating end-of-life care. In fact, all the major world religions accept end-of-life care when the decision is made by a team of senior physicians, rather than just by one physician alone. In the case of Muslims, Islam says that you must do everything possible to continue life even when it has become futile; however, there are many *fatwas* that state that end-of-life decisions are acceptable, in accordance with Islam and best made by the medical. However, Article 63 of the Islamic Code of Medical Ethics could be regarded as a clarion call on Muslim medical personnel[7]. The Article states that "the treatment of a patient can be terminated if a team of medical experts or a medical committee involved in the management of such patient are satisfied that the continuation of treatment would be futile or useless." It further states that "treatment of patients whose condition has been confirmed to be useless by the medical committee should not be commenced."

Some of these *fatwas* go beyond the introduction of a non-escalation of care policy, and discuss the withdrawal of life support, which is venturing into the unethical territory and not usually practiced in Western medicine[8].

Disagreement between the Medical Team and the Family on End-of-Life Care

If communication has been good and trust has been established between the family and the medical team, there would not be a conflict when the medical team decides to implement end-of-life care. Therefore, the decision-making would have been over a period rather than a single abrupt event.

The agreement should be obtained in the following ways:

- ➤ The family should be encouraged to discuss the issue with friends or acquaintances who have medical knowledge.
- ➤ The family should be encouraged to read known publications on the issue. Medical Councils and Colleges of Physicians produce such documents.
- ➤ The family should be free to ask questions at their daily meetings with the medical team.
- ➤ It should be emphasized throughout that the decision to implement end-of-life care is the decision of the entire medical team and not the decision of just one person, however senior.
- ➤ The family should be reminded that the decision and implementation of end-of-life care are in accordance with hospital policy, see King Hamad University Hospital End-of-Life Care Policy, Appendix A.

If a family does not agree with the implementation of end-of-life care in spite of all the above, it is important that there is an authority beyond the ICU to which the family could appeal to. Most hospitals have an Ethics Committee, and the family should be referred to the Ethics Committee to discuss the issue further. The Ethics Committee has the advantage of not being involved with the patient on a day-to-day basis and could maintain a more detached and balanced view. It would normally consist of both practicing physicians and lay people.

The ICU team should cooperate with the decision of the Ethics Committee, even when they disagree with it.

Advance Directives

Advance directives are now commonplace internationally. A patient writes down what aspects of treatment he would like or not like to receive in the event he is unable to make decisions in the future.

It is signed and witnessed and available to place in the patient's file. A physician could talk to the patient and obtain the patient's instructions face-to-face and know what the patient would or would not consent to. The problem arises when a patient is in the ICU and unable to discuss face-to-face the directives with the ICU physicians. Advance directives are not legally recognized in all jurisdictions.

An alternative but similar option is a healthcare proxy where a person authorizes a friend or relative to make decisions on their behalf if they become incapacitated.

Physicians should be certain of their legal ground before agreeing to follow an advance directive or health care proxy. If in doubt, it is advised to follow international standards of end-of-life care and refer the matter to the Hospital Ethics Committee.

Consolidating End-of-Life Care Strategies

There is a need to educate the public, and indeed the medical profession about end-of-life care strategies. If people are educated about the issue, they would understand the complexity of the subject, the strategies and the ethics of the situation. In Australia, the Queensland government has published a statewide strategy for end-of-life care in all areas of medical care[9]. It has outlined four main areas:

- ➢ Expand the knowledge of end-of-life care and create a comprehensive awareness. Ensure education of the public and public health organizations of the benefits of planning and delivery of end-of-life care.
- ➢ Ensure that the earliest possible identification of patients who would or are anticipated to have shortened life expectancy as a result of known health conditions is routinely achieved, together with timely Advanced Care Planning (ACP) and the initiation of coordinated planning of end-of-life care.

> Ensure that end-of-life-care delivered in public services consistently responds to the needs of patients and meets established clinical safety and quality standards.
> Ensure that the strategic capability and configuration of end-of-life care services is strengthened to maximize system health service delivery and performance.

The UK government has declared its commitment to delivering high-quality end-of-life care in a document published in July 2015. It promised to improve the quality of care, appoint end-of-life care commissioners locally, put the right clinicians with the right skills in place and to strengthen accountability and transparency in the area of end-of-life care[10].

CONCLUSION

The international drive for improving end-of-life care seems to be unstoppable in encouraging education of both physicians and the public.

REFERENCES

1. Tierney E, Kauts V. Do Not Resuscitate [DNR] Policies in the ICU – the Time Has Come for Openness and Change. Bah Med Bull 2014; 36(2): 65-8.
2. Ismail M, Khashaba S Elmusharaf K, et al. Misunderstanding of the Term "DNR" in a Middle-Eastern Teaching Hospital. Bah Med Bull 2015; 37(2): 88-91.
3. American College of Surgeons. Advanced Trauma Life Support Provider Manual. 8th ed. Chicago: American College of Surgeons, 2008. http://www.fracturedpublisher.com/advanced-trauma-life-support-manual-american.pdf. Accessed in July 2016
4. Rabkin MT, Gillerman G, Rice NR. Orders Not to Resuscitate. N Engl J Med 1976; 295(7): 364-6.
5. Pontoppidan H, Abbott WM, Brewster DC, et al. Optimum Care for Hopelessly Ill Patients — A Report of the Clinical Care

Committee of the Massachusetts General Hospital. N Engl J Med 1976; 295(7): 362-4.
6. Donnelly L. 'Unforgivable' Failings in End-of-Life Care Revealed as 40,000 Dying Patients Subject to Secret 'Do Not Resuscitate' Orders Every Year. The Telegraph 2016. http://www.telegraph.co.uk/news/2016/05/01/unforgivable-failings-in-end-of-life-care-revealed-40000-dying-p/ Accessed July 2016.
7. International Conference on Islamic Medicine. The Islamic Code of Medical Ethics. Kuwait, 1981. http://www.encyclopedia.com/science/encyclopedias-almanacs-transcripts-and-maps/islamic-code-medical-ethics-kuwait-document. Accessed July 2016.
8. Administration of Islamic Research and Ifta. Fatwa No. 12086. Riyadh, Kingdom of Saudi Arabia, 1988.
9. Statewide Health Service Strategy and Planning Unit, Health Commissioning Queensland. Statewide Strategy for End-Of-Life-Care. State of Queensland: Queensland Health, 2015.
10. National Health Services Finance and Operations. Our Commitment to You for End-Of-Life Care: The Government Response to the Review of Choice in End of Life. London, United Kingdom: Crown, 2015. https://www.gov.uk/government/uploads/system/uploads/attachment_data/file/ 536326/choice-response.pdf. Accessed July 2016.

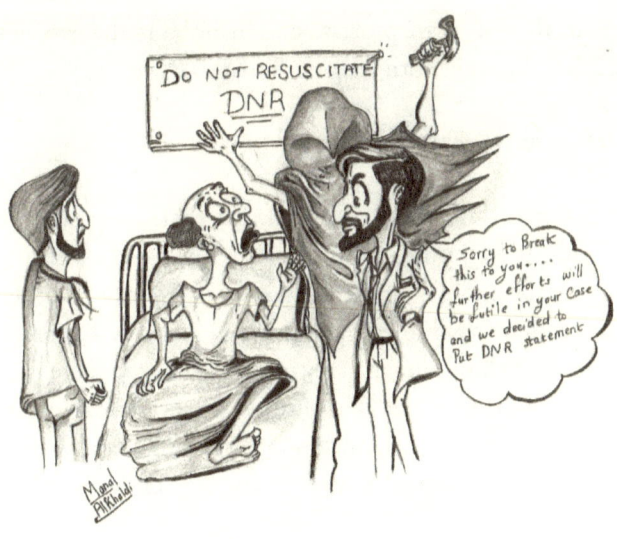

Appendix A - Summary

1. **Policy Purpose**

    1.1. This document aims to set out guidelines to facilitate the appropriate issuing of End-of-Life Care orders.

2. **Detailed Policy Statement**

    2.1. This policy is applicable to adult and pediatric patients in all areas of the hospital.
    2.2. This policy is designed to understand and articulate the desirable outcomes of care so that health care teams can limit interventions including cardiopulmonary resuscitation and renal replacement therapy that are not consistent with the goals of care. The processes and outcomes involved in meeting the goals of care should be:
    2.2.1. Medically appropriate. 2.2.2. Ethically permissible.
    2.2.3. Respectful of patients' values and cultures.
    2.2.4. Delivered in a way that will promote comfort and dignity, meet family's needs for privacy, grieving, and spirituality.
    2.2.5. Respectful of the complementary roles and perspectives of all health care professionals involved in the patient's care.
    2.2.6. Consistent with religious jurisprudence.

3. **Definitions**

    3.1. End-of-Life Care status means that no procedures for advanced resuscitation are to be initiated, such as chest compressions, defibrillation, cardioversion, intubation/ventilation, advanced cardiac life support (ACLS) procedures and medications, and continuous renal replacement therapy (unless the patient is in chronic kidney disease and already on intermittent hemodialysis). All other supportive measures, including nursing, physiotherapy, all comfort medications, antibiotics, etc. will continue. End-of-Life Care status applies solely to cardiopulmonary and renal resuscitation, such as all artificial mechanical and electrical means of support and vasopressor and inotropic support.

3.2. It should be made clear to all staff and the patient's relatives that all other treatments and care that are appropriate for the patient are not excluded and should not be influenced by an End-of-Life Care order.

3.3. An End-of-Life Care decision is different from "Non-escalation of Care" or "Non-escalation of treatment". Non-escalation of care or Non-escalation of treatment is a decision not to add more complex care/treatment in a situation where a patient is already receiving care/treatment but is not responding. This decision is a matter of clinical judgment on the part of an attending team and it is already a part of routine clinical practice, such as when a surgeon determines that surgery is futile or when an oncologist determines that further chemotherapy is futile.

4. Areas of Responsibility

4.1. Consultants Involved:

4.1.1. The attending consultant will consider the issue of End-of-Life Care in the initial assessment of all newly admitted patients and where it is appropriate will be pro-active in initiating End-of-Life Care before complex treatment begins.

4.1.2. The attending consultant (or the consultant intensivist if the patient is in ICU/the ED consultant if the patient is in the ED) is responsible to determine the End-of-Life Care decision and to appoint a team of two consultants, which may include the attending consultant or ICU consultant/ ED consultant himself/herself to make the End-of-Life Care decision.

4.1.3. The team of two consultants will assess the patient, make a decision, and write it in the patient's documentation.

4.1.4. It is the responsibility of the health care team involved in the patient's care to be aware of the End-of-Life Care decision.

4.2. Resuscitation/Ethics Committee:

4.2.1. It is the responsibility of the Resuscitation/Ethics Committee to provide consultancy with regards to End-of-Life Care decisions in an advisory capacity.

5. Procedures for Implementation

5.1. All patients will be fully resuscitated unless End-of-Life Care is agreed by the attending team and signed by two consultants in the patient's electronic file.

5.2. The responsibility of identifying the patient in whom End-of-Life Care status is appropriate is that of the treating consultant at that point in time in consultation with another consultant, in agreement with the health care team and other allied team members. End-of-Life Care is a team decision rather than an individual one. The primary consultant (or consultant intensivist if the patient is in ICU/the ED consultant if the patient is in ED) will solicit the opinion of two teams concerning the End-of-Life Care status of the patient who fits the description of the item above. Ideally, but not always, the two team consultants should comprise the admitting consultant and another consultant in the same specialty. In ICU the consultants should be an ICU consultant and an admitting team consultant. In ED the consultants should be an ED consultant and an admitting team consultant.

5.3. The circumstances in which the two consultants can sign an End-of-Life Care order are as follows:

5.3.1. The two teams agree that the patient is not medically fit for resuscitation.

5.3.2. The two teams decide that cardiopulmonary and renal resuscitation are futile and inappropriate for a specific situation, irrespective of the opinion of the patient or the patient's relatives.

5.3.3. The two consultants enter a note in the chart as follows: (an example) "In my opinion ACLS resuscitation measures and renal replacement therapy (RRT) will not benefit the patient and should not be carried out."

5.3.4. It is not sufficient to write "Not for Ventilation" as ventilation is only one of many ACLS measures. The note should always specify the terms ACLS and RRT.

5.3.5. A patient on whom an End-of-Life Care order has been written should not be admitted to the ICU as the complex care provided in ICU will not be appropriate.

5.3.6. In circumstances where a consultant is not immediately available a senior registrar may sign the End-of-Life Care order on his/her behalf, provided that the senior registrar records that the responsible consultant has agreed by telephone that the End-of-Life Care order is appropriate, and that the consultant confirms the End-of-Life Care order in the patient file within 24 hours.

5.4. A mentally competent patient who has the capacity to consent has the right to refuse resuscitation as long as he/she is fully informed regarding the implications of his/her choices. Initiation of resuscitation against the patient's wishes violates an individual's rights to self-determination and death with dignity.

5.5. The following listed conditions are some examples, among others, of situations where End-of-Life Care should be initiated, and the decision to initiate End-of-Life Care is a matter of the two consultants' judgment:

5.5.1. Advanced incurable malignancy

5.5.2. Advanced multi-organ failure

5.5.3. Severe, well-documented brain damage

5.5.4. Advanced cardiac or pulmonary disease not amenable to treatment 5.5.5. Inoperable congenital heart disease

5.5.6. Fatal chromosomal or neuromuscular disease

5.5.7. Severe mental or physical incapacity in addition to other major co-existing illness. 5.5.8. Brain death (due to any etiology), once declared according to established policy, and if organ donation is not planned.

5.6. End-of-Life Care order should only be implemented in a situation where full information is available to the teams. For example, in the Emergency Department, if information is not available, then an End-of-Life Care order cannot be given. However, if there is time to obtain full information on the patient's overall condition, then that information should be obtained quickly.

5.7. End-of-Life Care must be explained to the patient or the patient's family in understandable terms indicating the futility of medical intervention in the patient's care, and this should be documented. If a family is not contactable in person or by telephone after at least three attempts over a period of a minimum of one hour, then End-of-Life Care Decisions can be implemented without informing the family.

5.8. It is necessary only to inform the patient or the patient's family of the End-of-Life Care decision rather than seek their involvement and consent in the End-of-Life Care decision.

5.9. In the case of Muslim patients, the Islamic religion's concepts concerning End-of-Life decisions have been clarified by the Presidency of the Administration of Islamic Research and Ifta, Riyadh, KSA, in their Fatwa No. 12086 issued on 30.6.1409 (Hijra) [1988 (AD)]. The Fatwa allows a decision not to apply resuscitation where it will not benefit the patient. It specifically mentions that there is no need to use resuscitators in "obstinate, incurable illness, untreatable brain damage after suffering heart or lung failure for the first time, a state of mental inactivity due to a chronic illness, an advanced stage of cancer, a chronic heart or lung illness, or the recurrence of heart and lungs failure."

5.9.1. In addition, regarding family involvement, The Fatwa states that: "No consideration should be given to the opinion of the patient's family as to whether or not resuscitation should be applied because this is not their area of expertise."

5.10. In the event where the patient or the patient's family insists on implementing cardiopulmonary resuscitation to the patient, the primary consultant should involve the second consultant to meet the family and inform the family of the situation. If there is still no acceptance, then the matter should be referred to the Resuscitation Committee or Ethics Committee.

5.11. The patient's legal representative, for minor or incompetent patients, has the right to refuse resuscitation, if their decision is medically sound and represents the best interest of the patient, as long as they are fully informed regarding the implications of their choices.

5.12. Documentation of End-of-Life Care order:

5.12.1. The End-of-Life Care status shall be reviewed by the attending consultant (or consultant intensivist/ED consultant) at two-weekly intervals, and where there are changes in the patient's condition. The review intervals shall be noted in the patient's medical record.

5.12.2. The orders for End-of-Life Care should be agreed by the medical team and entered by the two consultants or senior registrars directly and personally on the patient's electronic record, not through a senior house officer or a registrar.

5.12.3. Once the patient is discharged from King Hamad University Hospital, the End-of-Life Care status is not valid.

5.12.4. Inform the following personnel of the decision:

5.12.4.1. Physicians
5.12.4.2. Nursing Staff
5.12.4.3. Patient relatives and patient (if appropriate)

5.12.4.4. Future care providers (when transferred to other wards)

5.12.5. Patient's legal representative:

The patient's legal representative is a person authorized by law to make treatment decisions for an incompetent or under-aged patient, and shall be given deference in the following order:

5.12.5.1. Legal guardian
5.12.5.2. Husband
5.12.5.3. Father
5.12.5.4. Other male relative
5.12.5.5. Mother
5.12.5.6. Other female relative

REFERENCES

1. Campbell ML. Forgoing Life-Sustaining Therapy: How to Care for the Patient Who is Near Death. American Association of Critical Care Nurses 1998: 140.
2. von Gunten CF, Ferris FD, Emanuel LL. The Patient-Physician Relationship. Ensuring Competency in End-of-Life Care: Communication and Relational Skills. JAMA 2000; 284(23):3051-7.
3. Kitchens LW, Brennan TA, Carroll RJ, et al. Ethics Manual: Fourth Edition. Ann Intern Med 1998; 128(7):576-594.
4. Appelbaum PS. Clinical Practice. Assessment of Patients' Competence to Consent to Treatment. N Engl J Med 2007; 357(18):1834-40.
5. General Medical Council. Withholding and Withdrawing - Guidance for Doctors. http://www.gmc-uk.org/Withholding_and_withdrawing_guidance_for_doctors.pdf_33377901.pdf
6. Presidency of the Administration of Islamic Research and Ifta, Riyadh, KSA
   Fatwa No. 12086 issued on 30.6.1409 (Hijra) [1988 (AD)].

ETHICAL STANDARDS IN PSYCHIATRIC PRACTICE

King Hamad University Hospital adopts the World Psychiatric Association - Madrid Declaration on Ethical Standards for Psychiatric Practice. The Madrid Declaration on Ethical Standards for Psychiatric Practice published in the website of World Psychiatric Association (WPA) is an excellent guideline to be followed in research and in dealing with other psychiatric issues.

Madrid Declaration on Ethical Standards for Psychiatric Practice

Approved by the General Assembly of the World Psychiatric Association in Madrid, Spain, on August 25, 1996, and enhanced by the WPA General Assemblies in Hamburg, Germany on August 8, 1999, in Yokohama, Japan, on August 26, 2002, in Cairo, Egypt, on September 12, 2005, and in Buenos Aires, Argentina, on September 21, 2011.

DECLARATION OF MADRID

In 1977, the World Psychiatric Association approved the Declaration of Hawaii which set out ethical guidelines for the practice of psychiatry. The Declaration was updated in Vienna in 1983. To reflect the impact of changing social attitudes and new medical developments on the psychiatric profession, the World Psychiatric Association has once again undertaken a review of ethical standards that should be abided to by all its members and all persons practicing psychiatry.

Medicine is both a healing art and a science. The dynamics of this combination are best reflected in psychiatry, the branch of medicine that specializes in the care and protection of those who are ill or infirm, because of a mental disorder or impairment. Although there may be cultural, social and national differences, the need for ethical conduct and continual review of ethical standards is universal.

As practitioners of medicine, psychiatrists must be aware of the ethical implications of being a physician, and of the specific ethical demands of the specialty of psychiatry. As members of society, psychiatrists must advocate for fair and equal treatment of the mentally ill, for social justice and equity for all.

Ethical practice is based on the psychiatrist's individual sense of responsibility to the patient and judgment in determining what is correct and appropriate conduct. External standards and influences such as professional codes of conduct, the study of ethics, or the rule of law by themselves will not guarantee the ethical practice of medicine.

Psychiatrists should keep in mind at all times the boundaries of the psychiatrist-patient relationship, and be guided primarily by the respect for patients and concern for their welfare and integrity.

It is in this spirit that the World Psychiatric Association approved at the General Assembly on August 25th, 1996, amended on August 8th 1999 and on August 26th 2002 the following ethical standards that should govern the practice of psychiatrists universally.

1. Psychiatry is a medical discipline concerned with the prevention of mental disorders in the population, the provision of the best possible treatment for mental disorders, the rehabilitation of

individuals suffering from mental illness and the promotion of mental health. Psychiatrists serve patients by providing the best therapy available consistent with accepted scientific knowledge and ethical principles. Psychiatrists should devise therapeutic interventions that are least restrictive to the freedom of the patient and seek advice in areas of their work about which they do not have primary expertise. While doing so, psychiatrists should be aware of and concerned with the equitable allocation of health resources.

2. It is the duty of psychiatrists to keep abreast of scientific developments of the specialty and to convey updated knowledge to others. Psychiatrists trained in research should seek to advance the scientific frontiers of psychiatry.

3. The patient should be accepted as a partner by right in the therapeutic process. The psychiatrist-patient relationship must be based on mutual trust and respect to allow the patient to make free and informed decisions. It is the duty of psychiatrists to provide the patient with all relevant information so as to empower the patient to come to a rational decision according to personal values and preferences.

4. When the patient is gravely disabled, incapacitated and/or incompetent to exercise proper judgment because of a mental disorder, the psychiatrists should consult with the family and, if appropriate, seek legal counsel, to safeguard the human dignity and the legal rights of the patient. No treatment should be provided against the patient's will, unless withholding treatment would endanger the life of the patient and/or the life of others. Treatment must always be in the best interest of the patient.

5. When psychiatrists are requested to assess a person, it is their duty first to inform and advise the person being assessed about the purpose of the intervention, the use of the findings, and the possible repercussions of the assessment. This is particularly important when psychiatrists are involved in third party situations.

6. Information obtained in the therapeutic relationship is private to the patient and should be kept in confidence and used, only and exclusively, for the purpose of improving the mental health of the patient. Psychiatrists are prohibited from making use of such information for personal reasons, or personal benefit. Breach of confidentiality may only be appropriate when required by law (as in obligatory reporting of child abuse) or when serious physical or mental harm to the patient or to a third person would ensue if confidentiality were maintained; whenever possible, psychiatrists should first advise the patient about the action to be taken.
7. Research that is not conducted in accordance with the canons of science and that is not scientifically valid is unethical. Research activities should be approved by an appropriately constituted ethics committee. Psychiatrists should follow national and international rules for the conduct of research. Only individuals properly trained for research should undertake or direct it. Because psychiatric patients constitute a particularly vulnerable research population, extra caution should be taken to assess their competence to participate as research subjects and to safeguard their autonomy and their mental and physical integrity. Ethical standards should also be applied in the selection of population groups, in all types of research including epidemiological and sociological studies and in collaborative research involving other disciplines or several investigating centres.

GUIDELINES CONCERNING SPECIFIC SITUATIONS

The World Psychiatric Association Ethics Committee recognizes the need to develop a number of specific guidelines on a number of specific situations. The first five were approved by the General Assembly in Madrid, Spain, on August 25, 1996, the 6 through 8 by the General Assembly in Hamburg, Germany, on August 8, 1999, the 9 through 12 by the General Assembly in Yokohama, Japan, on

August 26, 2002, the 13 through 15 at the General Assembly in Cairo, Egypt, on September 12, 2005, and the 16 at the General Assembly in Buenos Aires, Argentina, on September 21, 2011.

1. Euthanasia:

A physician's duty, first and foremost, is the promotion of health, the reduction of suffering, and the protection of life. The psychiatrist, among whose patients are some who are severely incapacitated and incompetent to reach an informed decision, should be particularly careful of actions that could lead to the death of those who cannot protect themselves because of their disability. The psychiatrist should be aware that the views of a patient may be distorted by mental illness such as depression. In such situations, the psychiatrist's role is to treat the illness.

2. Torture:

Psychiatrists shall not take part in any process of mental or physical torture, even when authorities attempt to force their involvement in such acts.

3. Death Penalty:

Under no circumstances should psychiatrists participate in legally authorized executions nor participate in assessments of competency to be executed.

4. Selection of Sex:

Under no circumstances should a psychiatrist participate in decisions to terminate pregnancy for the purpose of sex selection.

5. Organ Transplantation:

The role of the psychiatrist is to clarify the issues surrounding organ donations and to advise on religious, cultural, social and family factors to ensure that informed and proper decisions be made by all concerned. The psychiatrists should not act as a proxy decision maker for patients nor use psychotherapeutic skills to influence the decision of a patient in these matters. Psychiatrists should seek to protect their patients and help them exercise self-determination to the fullest extent possible in situations of organ transplantation.

6. Psychiatrists addressing the media:

In all contacts with the media psychiatrists shall ensure that people with mental illness are presented in a manner which preserves their dignity and pride, and which reduces stigma and discrimination against them.

An important role of psychiatrists is to advocate for those people who suffer from mental disorders. As the public perception of psychiatrists and psychiatry reflects on patients, psychiatrists shall ensure that in their contact with the media they represent the profession of psychiatry with dignity.

Psychiatrists shall not make announcements to the media about presumed psychopathology on any individuals.

In presenting research findings to the media, psychiatrists shall ensure the scientific integrity of the information given and be mindful of the potential impact of their statements on the public perception of mental illness and on the welfare of people with mental disorders.

7. Psychiatrists and discrimination on ethnic or cultural grounds:

Discrimination by psychiatrists on the basis of ethnicity or culture, whether directly or by aiding others is unethical. Psychiatrists shall never be involved or endorse, directly or indirectly, any activity related to ethnic cleansing.

8. Psychiatrists and genetic research and counseling:

Research on the genetic bases of mental disorders is rapidly increasing and more people suffering from mental illness are participating in such research.

Psychiatrists involved in genetic research or counseling shall be mindful of the fact that the implication of genetic information are not limited to the individual from whom it was obtained and that its disclosure can have negative and disruptive effects on the families and communities of the individuals concerned.

Psychiatrist shall therefore ensure that:

- People and families who participate in genetic research do so with a fully informed consent;
- Any genetic information in their possession is adequately protected against unauthorized access, misinterpretation or misuse;
- Care is taken in communication with patients and families to make clear that current genetic knowledge is incomplete and may be altered by future findings. Psychiatrists shall only refer people to facilities for diagnostic genetic testing if that facility has:
- Demonstrated satisfactory quality assurance, procedures for such testing;
- Adequate and easily accessible resources for genetic counseling.

Genetic counseling with regard to family planning or abortion shall be respectful of the patients' value system, while providing sufficient medical and psychiatric information to aid patients make decisions they consider best for them.

9. Ethics of Psychotherapy in Medicine:

Medical treatments of any nature should be administered under the provisions of good practice guidelines regarding their indications, effectiveness, safety, and quality control. Psychotherapy, in its broadest sense, is an accepted component of many medical interactions. In a more specific and restricted sense, psychotherapy utilizes techniques involving verbal and non-verbal communication and interaction to achieve specified treatment goals in the care of specific disorders. Psychiatrists providing specific forms of psychotherapy must have appropriate training in such techniques. The general guidelines that apply to any medical treatment also apply to specific forms of psychotherapy in regard to its indications and outcomes, positive or negative. The effectiveness of psychotherapy and its place in a treatment plan are important subjects for both researchers and clinicians.

Psychotherapy by psychiatrists is a form of treatment for mental and other illnesses and emotional problems. The treatment approach utilized is determined in concert by the doctor and patient and/or the patient's family and/or guardians following a careful history and examination employing all relevant clinical and laboratory studies. The approach employed should be specific to the disease and patient's needs and sensitive to personal, familial, religious and cultural factors. It should be based on sound research and clinical wisdom and have the purpose of removing, modifying or retarding symptoms or disturbed patterns of behavior. It should promote positive adaptations including personal growth and development.

Psychiatrists and other clinicians responsible for a patient have to ensure that these guidelines are fully applied. Therefore, the psychiatrist or other delegated qualified clinician should determine the indications for psychotherapy and follow its development. In this context the essential notion is that the treatment is the consequence of a diagnosis and both are medical acts performed to take care of an ill person. These two levels of decisions, interventions and responsibilities are similar to other situations in clinical medicine; however, this does not exclude other interventions such as rehabilitation, which can be administered by non-medical personnel.

1. Like any other treatment in medicine, the prescription of psychotherapy should follow accepted guidelines for obtaining informed consent prior to the initiation of treatment as well as updating it in the course of treatment if goals and objectives of treatment are modified in a significant way.
2. If clinical wisdom, long standing and well-established practice patterns (this takes into consideration cultural and religious issues) and scientific evidence suggest potential clinical benefits to combining medication treatment with psychotherapy this should be brought to the patient's attention and fully discussed.
3. Psychotherapy explores intimate thoughts, emotions and fantasies, and as such may engender intense transference and counter-transference. In a psychotherapy relationship the power is unequally shared between the therapist and patient, and under no circumstances shall the psychotherapist use this relationship to personal advantage or transgress the boundaries established by the professional relationship.
4. At the initiation of psychotherapy, the patient shall be advised that information shared and health records will be kept in confidence except where the patient gives specific informed consent for release of information to third parties, or where a court order may require the production of records. The other exception is where there is a legal requirement to report certain information as in the case of child abuse.

10. Conflict of Interest in Relationship with Industry:

Although most organizations and institutions, including the WPA, have rules and regulations governing their relationship with industry and donors, individual physicians are often involved in interactions with the pharmaceutical industry, or other granting agencies that could lead to ethical conflict. In these situations, psychiatrists should be mindful of and apply the following guidelines.

1. The practitioner must diligently guard against accepting gifts that could have an undue influence on professional work.
2. Psychiatrists conducting clinical trials are under an obligation to disclose to the Ethics Review Board and their research subjects their financial and contractual obligations and benefits related to the sponsor of the study. Every effort should be made to set up review boards composed of researchers, ethicists and community representatives to assure the rights of research subjects are protected.
3. Psychiatrists conducting clinical trials have to ensure that their patients have understood all aspects of the informed consent. The level of education or sophistication of the patient is no excuse for bypassing this commitment. If the patient is deemed incompetent the same rules would apply in obtaining informed consent from the substitute decision maker. Psychiatrists must be cognizant that covert commercial influence on the trial design, promotion of drugs trials without scientific value, breach of confidentiality, and restrictive contractual clauses regarding publication of results may each in different ways encroach upon the freedom of science and scientific information.

11. Conflicts Arising with Third Party Players:

The obligations of organizations toward shareholders or the administrator regarding maximization of profits and minimization of costs can be in conflict with the principles of good practice. Psychiatrists working in such potentially conflicting environments, should uphold the rights of the patients to receive the best treatment possible.

1. In agreement with the UN Resolution 46/119 of the "Principles for the Protection of Persons with Mental Illness", psychiatrists should oppose discriminatory practices which limit their benefits and entitlements, deny parity curb the scope of treatment, or limit their access to proper medications for patients with a mental disorder.
2. Professional independence to apply best practice guidelines and clinical wisdom in upholding the welfare of the patient should be the primary considerations for the psychiatrist. It is also the duty of the psychiatrist to protect the patient privacy and confidentiality as part of preserving the sanctity and healing potential of the doctor-patient relationship.

12. Violating the Clinical Boundaries and Trust between Psychiatrists and Patients:

The psychiatrist-patient relationship may be the only relationship that permits an exploration of the deeply personal and emotional space, as granted by the patient. Within this relationship, the psychiatrist's respect for the humanity and dignity of the patient builds a foundation of trust that is essential for a comprehensive treatment plan. The relationship encourages the patient to explore deeply held strengths, weaknesses, fears, and desires, and many of these might be related to sexuality. Knowledge of these characteristics of the patient places the psychiatrist in a position of advantage that the patient allows on the expectation of trust and respect. Taking advantage of that knowledge by manipulating the patient's sexual fears and desires in order to obtain sexual access is a breach of the trust, regardless of consent. In the therapeutic relationship, consent on the part of the patient is considered vitiated by the knowledge the psychiatrist possesses about the patient and by the power differential that vests the psychiatrist with special authority over the patient. Consent under these circumstances will be tantamount to exploitation of the patient.

The latent sexual dynamics inherent in all relationships can become manifest in the course of the therapeutic relationship and if they are not properly handled by the therapist can produce anguish to the patient. This anguish is likely to become more pronounced if seductive statements and inappropriate non-verbal behavior are used by the therapist. Under no circumstances, therefore, should a psychiatrist get involved with a patient in any form of sexual behavior, irrespective of whether this behavior is initiated by the patient or the therapist.

13. Protection of the Rights of Psychiatrists:

1. Psychiatrists need to protect their right to live up to the obligations of their profession and to the expectations the public has of them to treat and to advocate for the welfare of their patients.
2. Psychiatrists ought to have the right to practice their specialty at the highest level of excellence by providing independent assessments of a persons' mental condition and by instituting effective treatment and management protocols in accordance to best practices and evidence-based medicine.
3. There are aspects in the history of psychiatry and in present working expectations in some totalitarian political regimes and profit driven economical systems that increase psychiatrists' vulnerabilities to be abused in the sense of having to acquiesce to inappropriate demands to provide inaccurate psychiatric reports that help the system, but damage the interests of the person being assessed.
4. Psychiatrists also share the stigma of their patients and, similarly, can become victims of discriminatory practices.

It should be the right and the obligation of psychiatrists to practice their profession and to advocate for the medical needs and the social and political rights of their patients without suffering being outcast by the profession, being ridiculed in the media or persecuted.

14. Disclosing the Diagnosis of Alzheimer's Disease (AD) and Other Dementias:

AD patient's right to know is now a well-established priority, recognised by healthcare professionals. Most patients want all information available and to be actively involved in making decision about treatments. At the same time, patients have the right also not to know if that is their wish. All must be given the opportunity to learn as much or as little as they want to know.

The alteration of patient's cognition makes the ability to make judgements and insight more difficult. Patients with dementia are also often brought by family members which introduces into the doctor-patient relationship a third partner.

Doctors, patients and families who share the responsibilities for fighting and coping with Alzheimer's disease for years all require access to information on the disease, including the diagnosis.

In addition to the "patient's right to know", telling the patient has many benefits. Patients and/or families should be told the diagnosis as early as possible in the disease process. Having family (or informal carer) involved in the discussion of the disclosure process is highly beneficial.

The physician should give accurate and reliable information, using simple language. He also should assess the patient's and the family's understanding of the situation. As usual, the bad news should be accompanied by information on a treatment and management plan.

Information on physical or speech therapy, support groups, day care centres, and other interventions should be provided. It should also be emphasised that a reorganised family network can alleviate the carer's burden and maintain quality of life as far as possible.

There are some exceptions, some of them transitory, to the disclosure of the diagnosis to a patient with dementia: **(1)** severe dementia where understanding the diagnosis is unlikely; **(2)** when a phobia about the condition is likely, or **(3)** when a patient is severely depressed;

15. Dual Responsibilities of Psychiatrists:

These situations may arise as part of legal proceedings (i.e. fitness to stand trial, criminal responsibility, dangerousness, testamentary capacity) or other competency related needs, such as for insurance purposes when evaluating claims for benefits, or for employment purposes when evaluating fitness to work or suitability for a particular employment or specific task.

During therapeutic interactions conflicting situations may arise if the physician's knowledge of the patient's condition cannot be kept private or when clinical notes or medical records are part of a larger employment dossier, hence not confidential to the clinical personnel in charge of the case (i.e. the military, correctional systems, medical services for employees of large corporations, treatment protocols paid by third parties).

It is the duty of a psychiatrist confronted with dual obligations and responsibilities at assessment time to disclose to the person being assessed the nature of the triangular relationship and the absence of a therapeutic doctor-patient relationship, besides the obligation to report to a third party even if the findings are negative and potentially damaging to the interests of the person under assessment. Under these circumstances, the person may choose not to proceed with the assessment.

Additionally, psychiatrists should advocate for separation of records and for limits to exposure of information such that only elements of information that are essential for purposes of the agency can be revealed.

16. Working with patients and carers

1. Legislation, policy and clinical practice relevant to the lives and care of people living with mental disorders, whenever possible, should be developed in collaboration with patients and carers.
2. The international psychiatric community should promote and support the development of patients' organizations and carers' organizations.
3. International and local psychiatric organizations, including WPA through its programs and member societies, are expected to seek the involvement of patients and carers in their activities where appropriate.
4. The best clinical care of any person in acute or rehabilitation situations is done in collaboration between the patient, the carers and the clinicians.
5. WPA member societies and other psychiatric organizations should collaborate with patients' organizations, carers' organizations and other community organizations to lobby governments for political will and action for better funding of services, community education and fighting stigma.
6. Each country needs specific guidelines in order to apply these recommendations.

REFERENCES

1. http://www.wpanet.org/detail.php?section_id=5&content_id=48. Accessed January 2017.

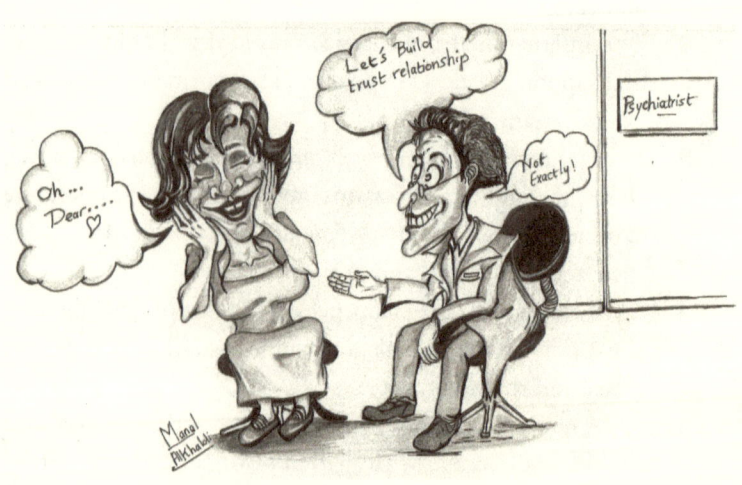

ETHICAL PERSPECTIVES IN ONCOLOGY PRACTICE

Elias Fadel

By definition, ethics (the Greek word "ethos" meaning "well-developed habits") is a branch of philosophy that involves systematizing, defending and recommending concepts of right and wrong conduct[1]. Ethics are moral principles that govern a person's behavior or conduct.

Oncology, on the other hand, is a branch of medicine that deals with the prevention, diagnosis and treatment of cancer.

An oncology practitioner (physician, nurse and paramedic) frequently confronts ethical issues during the daily practice, such as confidentiality, patient's right to access adequate care, informed consent, breaking bad news, allow natural death and so forth. In any situation, the code of ethics would be respected if the caregiver follows the framework of ethical reasoning called "principalism" which relies on four major guiding principles:

- ➢ Autonomy is the right for informed patients to participate in medical decision making.
- ➢ Beneficence mandates that clinicians are committed to act in the best interests of the patient.

> Non-maleficence demands that the health caregivers "do no harm".
> Justice requires that all people to be treated well and fairly, and health resources are used equitably.

Breaking Bad News

The bad news is defined as "if it drastically and negatively alters the patient's view of his/her future"[2].

Hippocrates encouraged physicians to "conceal most things from the patient while attending. Give necessary orders with cheerfulness and serenity, turning his attention away from what is being done to him; sometimes reprove sharply and emphatically, and sometimes comfort with solicitude and attention, revealing nothing of the patient's future or present condition"[3].

However, through the ages, and thanks to better education, more people would want to be autonomous in making their healthcare decisions, which demand an inevitable obligation from the healthcare giver to provide appropriate information to the patient[4].

In many Western countries, the majority of newly diagnosed patients with cancer would like to be informed about the potential effectiveness of treatment, its duration and its side effects[5-7]. However, a small percentage would like to know about their specific prognosis[6].

In the non-Western cultures, fewer than half of the patients are properly informed about their diagnosis, and a high percentage of patients would avoid discussion about the prognosis (>70%)[6]. Many factors contribute to this attitude[8-13].

> The perception that cancer is an incurable disease
> Social stigma related to cancer
> Family-centered model of decision-making

- The patient's family efforts to prevent the patient being informed because of the fear of a psychological breakdown and life-threatening reactions
- Language barrier
- Particular cultural values and beliefs

The following consensual principles for breaking bad news were developed through evidence review:

- "One person should be responsible for breaking bad news.
- The patient has a legal and moral right to information.
- The primary responsibility of the caregiver is to the patient.
- The person involved should be given accurate and reliable information.
- The persons involved should be asked how much they want to know.
- The person should be prepared for the possibility of bad news as early as possible in the diagnostic sequence.
- If several tests are being performed, avoid giving the results of each test individually.
- The person should be told the diagnosis as soon as it is certain and when the patient is ready.
- The person should be ensured of privacy and made to feel comfortable.
- Ideally, family and significant others should be present (if the patient allows).
- If possible, another health professional should be present.
- The patient's general practitioner and other medical advisers should be informed of the patient's situation and the level of understanding.
- Eye contact and body language should be used to convey warmth, empathy, encouragement or reassurance if culturally appropriate.
- If communication difficulties exist (e.g., hearing impairment, language differences), strategies should be adopted to address

these, such as the use of a trained health interpreter where language differences are evident.
➢ It is important to be sensitive to the person's culture, race, religious beliefs and social background.
➢ The clinicians breaking the bad news should acknowledge their shortcomings and emotional difficulties in undertaking the task."[14]

Breaking bad news is usually mediated through protocols of communication, such as the SPIKES, SHARE, ABCDE, GUIDE and BREAKS models[15,18-22].

The patient's perception of bad news depends on several factors, including:

➢ Patient's expectations
➢ Previous patient's experiences
➢ Patient's general personality and disposition
➢ Patient's beliefs and culture
➢ Physician attitude and communication skills
➢ Clarity and credibility of the provided information

However, as a general rule, physicians should promote hopefulness without endorsing unrealistic optimism[23].

Informed Consent

Informed consent is one of the patient rights and constitutes a fundamental principle of healthcare. It is a medico-legal process that involves effective physician-patient communication[24].

Three main historical turning points have led to the establishment of the patient's informed consent: the Nuremberg Code, the Declaration of Helsinki and the Belmont Report.

The Nuremberg Code was initiated after Nuremberg trials of the Nazi doctors' malpractices of inhuman experiments performed in the concentration camps[25]. The code was published in 1949 consisting of ten points, among them was the requirement of a "voluntary, well-informed consent of the human subject in a full legal capacity".

The Declaration of Helsinki was established in 1964; it includes ethical principles regarding human experimentation developed for the World Medical Association (WMA). The fundamental principle of the Declaration of Helsinki is the respect for the individual, the right to self-determination and the right to make informed decisions regarding participation in research[26].

The Belmont Report was issued on 30 September 1978 by the National Commission for the Protection of Human Subjects of Biomedical and Behavioral Research. It includes the principles of respect for persons, beneficence and justice[27]. Among the rules established by the US Congress based on the Belmont report was the creation of the Institutional Review Board (IRB), which reviews research proposals to determine if they are in line with the ethical code and thus, capable of being conducted.

The Good Clinical Practice (GCP) guidelines are international quality standards developed by the International Conference on Harmonization of Technical Requirements for Registration of Pharmaceuticals for Human Use. They include protection of rights and wellbeing of the subjects enrolled in a clinical trial.

The prelude for any patient's informed consent should include the following:

> ➤ Provide the patients with appropriate information regarding the nature of their disease, the treatment options and the prognosis.

- Confirm the patient's full understanding of the information delivered by asking the patient to recall and restate the key elements of the discussion.
- Ensure that the patients are mentally and psychologically capable of understanding and assimilating the information and taking a voluntary decision, whether by refusing or accepting a treatment or medical procedure that would affect their wellbeing.

Any health care intervention requires a patient's consent based on appropriate discussion, which includes, but is not limited to surgery, anesthesia, interventional diagnostic procedure, such as endoscopy or biopsy, radiation therapy, chemotherapy and blood tests, such as HIV testing.

The patient's acceptance is an inevitable prerequisite before the implementation of any treatment plan. However, informed consent is not required in case of emergency when delaying the treatment would put the patient at risk of a potential deleterious outcome.

The patient has the right to accept or reject a proposed treatment by his physician. The practice of paternalism by the healthcare providers has to be replaced by the inevitable requirement of obtaining 'informed consent' before proceeding with medical interventions[28].

However, the patient has no right to request medical intervention not indicated in his/her case, which is not based on the evidence-based medical practice[29].

In the case of a minor, the unconscious or the mentally incapable, a surrogate decision maker could be involved in approving the consent. The choice of surrogate depends on several factors:

- Family relationship
- Religion

- Culture
- National law/civil code

The healthcare team should confirm the authentic eligibility of the surrogate for this mission with an emphasis on honesty, impartiality, responsibility and respect of the patient's principles[30-31].

A competent patient could, in some communities, delegate a trusted relative to make treatment decisions.

Because children do not have the decision-making capacity to provide informed consent, the parents could sign on their behalf. The latter is to be distinguished from the informed consent which is given for an intervention for oneself.

The informed consent should in no way be considered as a defensive medico-legal document to make the healthcare provider immune against any future complaint by the patient. It is rather a proof that the physician exerted his/her obligation and duty towards their patient regarding engaging with a well-elaborated and oriented communication.

Effective physician-patient communication, according to some studies, could lead to better treatment outcomes and improved patient empowerment[32,33]. Other studies revealed that patient education could prevent potential medical errors and improve safety[34].

Do Not Resuscitate

Among the different ethical issues, the most critical that an oncologist could confront is the decision of "Do Not Resuscitate (DNR)", "Do Not Attempt Resuscitation (DNAR)" or "Allow Natural Death (AND)".

"The American Heart Association recommends that all patients in cardiac arrest should be resuscitated unless they have a valid Do Not

Resuscitate (DNR) order, or where resuscitation is physiologically futile (signs of irreversible death)"[35].

Only after a consensual and unanimous agreement by the involved physicians, would a patient become eligible to be declared as DNR. However, this would in no way abrogate the patient's right to accept or reject this decision.

The process of declaring a patient as DNR should abide by the following requirements:

- Medically confirmed hopeless condition based on the opinion of more than one qualified consultant (in general, three consultants)
- Thorough and fully transparent information to the patient or surrogate
- Witnessed acceptance of the patient or surrogate
- Implement the process of DNR according to pre-defined rules and regulations in line with the international standards
- Ensure that the patient rights are respected at all times

The physician's decision not to start CPR would be challenged by two concepts: the caregiver is committed not to harm others as by the principle of non-maleficence and not to engage in an aggressive intervention (CPR) knowing that it would cause harm to the patient whose imminent death cannot be prevented[36,37].

Many patients and relatives do not understand the purpose of DNR because of the fear that DNR would decrease the level of their care[38,39]. It is the doctor's responsibility to ensure that this does not happen. The care team has to assure the patient and relatives that DNR is implemented to protect the individual from unhelpful and potentially undignified treatment, while all other treatments needed for the comfort and dignity of the patient would be implemented[40].

The key ethical principles surrounding end-of-life decisions and resuscitation are[41]:

- Respect for autonomy: respect for individual liberty, values, beliefs and choices
- Beneficence: to do good and prevent or remove harm
- Non-maleficence: not to inflict harm or evil
- Justice: to treat patients equally

The core practical principles for end-of-life care are:

- Offer any medically acceptable therapy or measure which improves the quality of life
- Respect the dignity of both the patient and the caregiver
- Be sensitive to the patient's and family's wishes
- Assess and manage psychological, social, spiritual needs of the patient and his/her family
- Respect the physicians' decisions to limit their intervention or forgo any specific treatment which could be useless and probably harmful.

In general, if the patient refuses a DNR order, the doctor has no legal obligation to offer any treatment, which in his/her professional judgment would not be beneficial to the patient[40,42]. Attempting CPR in patients with end-stage cancer is medically inappropriate and promotes the myth that doctors could postpone death indefinitely. In general, given time and the opportunity for discussions, it is rare for a patient to continue to insist on attempts at resuscitation.

On the other hand, respect for autonomy restricts CPR application if the patient refuses it, but could not give the patient the right of CPR[40,43-44].

The patient's capacity to deal with the issue of DNR should be verified and, if necessary, assessed by a specialized practitioner. The patient should be able to understand and retain information about the decision and the consequences of having or not having the intervention.

If the patient is incompetent to make decisions, the family should be involved in discussions. The family should take into consideration the attitude the patient would have manifested if he/she was capable of taking a decision.

If a patient is incapable to make a decision or communicates his/her wish and in the absence of available relatives, the caregiver guided by Article 2 of the Human Rights Act 1998, would have the obligation of taking the decision in the patient's best interest. That is medical paternalism which conflicts with patient's autonomy defined as the human right for self-governance or self-determination[45]. Therefore, a healthcare practitioner who practices the medical paternalism requires a clear justification at all times[46].

Practitioners are expected to uphold and protect the patient's interests and well-being guided by the ethical principle of beneficence[47]. However, if a practitioner-led by the principles of honesty, facilitates a peaceful and dignified death of a hopeless condition, he could also be viewed as accomplishing a beneficent act.

Deontological ethics supports action as right if it accords with a moral rule irrespective of the outcome or the purpose; utilitarianism defines action as morally right if it produces good consequences[48].

From an Islamic perspective and according to some references, there is a consensus that DNR is acceptable in cases that meet the definition of death or in cases where three physicians have determined that the patient is terminally ill[49-53].

"The Presidency of the Administration of Islamic Research and Ifta, Riyadh, Kingdom of Saudi Arabia (KSA), in its Fatwa No. 12086 issued on 30.6.1409 (Hijra) [1988 (AD)], stated: If three knowledgeable and trustworthy physicians agreed that the patient's condition is hopeless, the life supporting machines can be withheld or withdrawn[51,54]." The family members' opinion is not included in decision making as they are unqualified to make such decision (translation by Takouri and Halawani)[51,54].

Euthanasia and Physician-Assisted Death

Euthanasia (from Greek "good death"), is the practice of intentionally ending a life to relieve pain and suffering. Mercy-killing is the term used in many countries and cultures.

Euthanasia may be classified as voluntary, non-voluntary or involuntary, according to whether the patient's informed consent has been obtained or not[55].

Involuntary euthanasia if performed on a person who is able to provide informed consent, but does not, either because they do not want to die or because they were not asked. **Non-voluntary euthanasia** or **mercy killing** is if performed when the consent of the individual is unavailable, such as in case of a persistent vegetative state, or young children.

Euthanasia used to be illegal worldwide, but it is being decriminalized under certain specific circumstances in many countries, such as in the Netherlands under the "Groningen Protocol"[56].

In euthanasia, the physician administers the means of death, usually by a lethal drug; in physician-assisted suicide (PAS), the patient administers the means of death.

The ethical reasons contradicting the legality of euthanasia and assisted death are medical and religious. The physician-assisted suicide is contrary to the original Hippocratic Oath of 400 BCE, stating "I will give no deadly medicine to anyone if asked, nor suggest any such counsel". The Declaration of Geneva, a revision of the Hippocratic Oath, first drafted in 1948 by the World Medical Association in response to euthanasia, eugenics and other medical crimes performed in Nazi Germany, contains[61], "I will maintain the utmost respect for human life". The International Code of Medical Ethics, last revised in 2006, states that "a physician shall always bear in mind the obligation to respect human life". Some religions, such as Islam, Christianity and Judaism are against euthanasia and physician-assisted death[57-61].

CONCLUSION

A healthcare practitioner must provide a compassionate voluntary treatment according to the International Gold Standards, while strictly abiding by the code of ethics, the patient's beliefs, cultures and will.

REFERENCES

1. Internet Encyclopaedia of Philosophy. www.iep.utm.edu/ethics/ Accessed on 17 March 2016.
2. Buckman R. Breaking Bad News: Why is it Still So Difficult? Br Med J (Clin Res Ed) 1984; 288(6430):1597-9.
3. Hippocrates. Decorum. In: Hippocrates, Jones WHS, et al, eds. 2nd ed. Cambridge: Harvard University Press, 1967: 297.
4. Sen M. Communication with Cancer Patients. The Influence of Age, Gender, Education, and Health Insurance Status. Ann N Y Acad Sci 1997; 809:514-24.
5. Rutten LJ, Arora NK, Bakos AD, et al. Information Needs and Sources of Information among Cancer Patients: A Systematic Review of Research (1980-2003). Patient Educ Couns 2005; 57(3):250-61.
6. Fujimori M, Uchitomi Y. Preferences of Cancer Patients Regarding Communication of Bad News: A Systematic Literature Review. Jpn J Clin Oncol 2009; 39(4):201-16.

7. Jenkins V, Fallowfield L, Saul J. Information Needs of Patients with Cancer: Results from a Large Study in UK Cancer Centres. Br J Cancer 2001; 84(1):48-51.
8. Bou Khalil R. Attitudes, Beliefs and Perceptions Regarding Truth Disclosure of Cancer-Related Information in the Middle East: A Review. Palliat Support Care 2013; 11(1):69-78.
9. Wuensch A, Tang L, Goelz T, et al. Breaking Bad News in China--The Dilemma of Patients' Autonomy and Traditional Norms. A First Communication Skills Training for Chinese Oncologists and Caretakers. Psychooncology 2013; 22(5):1192-5.
10. Back MF, Huak CY. Family Centred Decision Making and Non-Disclosure of Diagnosis in a South East Asian Oncology Practice. Psychooncology 2005; 14(12):1052-9.
11. Tse CY, Chong A, Fok SY. Breaking Bad News: A Chinese Perspective. Palliat Med 2003; 17(4):339-43.
12. Jiang Y, Liu C, Li JY, et al. Different Attitudes of Chinese Patients and Their Families toward Truth Telling of Different Stages of Cancer. Psychooncology 2007; 16(10):928-36.
13. Bousquet G, Orri M, Winterman S, et al. Breaking Bad News in Oncology: A Metasynthesis. J Clin Oncol 2015; 33(22):2437-43.
14. Girgis A, Sanson-Fisher RW. Breaking Bad News: Consensus Guidelines for Medical Practitioners. J Clin Oncol 1995; 13(9):2449-56.
15. Pang Y, Tang L, Zhang Y, et al. Breaking Bad News in China: Implementation and Comparison of Two Communication Skills Training Courses in Oncology. Psychooncology 2015; 24(5):608-11.
16. Fielding R, Hung J. Preferences for Information and Involvement in Decisions During Cancer Care among a Hong Kong Chinese Population. Psychooncology 1996; 5:321-9.
17. Costantini A, Baile WF, Lenzi R, et al. Overcoming Cultural Barriers to Giving Bad News: Feasibility of Training to Promote Truth-Telling to Cancer Patients. J Cancer Educ 2009; 24(3):180-5.
18. Tang WR, Chen KY, Hsu SH, et al. Effectiveness of Japanese SHARE Model in Improving Taiwanese Healthcare Personnel's Preference for Cancer Truth Telling. Psychooncology 2014; 23(3):259-65.

19. Baile WF, Buckman R, Lenzi R, et al. SPIKES-A Six-Step Protocol for Delivering Bad News: Application to the Patient with Cancer. Oncologist 2000; 5(4):302-11.
20. Rabow MW, McPhee SJ. Beyond Breaking Bad News: How to Help Patients Who Suffer. West J Med 1999; 171(4):260-3.
21. Narayanan V, Bista B, Koshy C. 'BREAKS' Protocol for Breaking Bad News. Indian J Palliat Care 2010; 16(2):61-5.
22. Back AL 2013 Vital Talk (1.0) [Mobile Application Software] http://vitaltalk.org Accessed on 13 January 2015.
23. Whitney SN, Mccullough LB, Frugé E, et al. Beyond Breaking Bad News: The Roles of Hope and Hopefulness. Cancer 2008; 113(2):442-5.
24. Salgo V. Leland Stanford Etc. Bd. Trustees. Court of Appeals of California. Docket No. 17045.
25. Annas GJ, Grodin MA. The Nazi Doctors and The Nuremberg Code. New York, NY: Oxford University Press Inc, 1992.
26. World Medical Association. Declaration of Helsinki: Ethical Principles for Medical Research Involving Human Subjects. JAMA 2013; 310(20): 2191-4.
27. National Commission for the Protection of Human Subjects of Biomedical and Behavioral Research, Department of Health, Education and Welfare. The Belmont Report. Washington, DC. https://videocast.nih.gov/pdf/ohrp_belmont_report.pdf
28. Katz J. The Silent World of Doctor and Patient. New York: The Free Press, 1984:23.
29. Cerminara KL. The Law and Its Interaction with Medical Ethics in End-of-Life Decision Making. Chest 2011; 140(3):775-80.
30. Pope TM. Legal Fundamentals of Surrogate Decision Making. Chest 2012; 141(4):1074-81.
31. Scheunemann LP, Arnold RM, White DB. The Facilitated Values History: Helping Surrogates Make Authentic Decisions for Incapacitated Patients with Advanced Illness. Am J Respir Crit Care Med 2012; 186(6):480-6.
32. Greenfield S, Kaplan S, Ware JE Jr. Expanding Patient Involvement in Care. Effects on Patient Outcomes. Ann Intern Med 1985; 102(4):520-8.
33. Stewart MA. Effective Physician-Patient Communication and Health Outcomes: A Review. CMAJ 1995; 152(9):1423-33.

34. Davis RE, Jacklin R, Sevdalis N, et al. Patient Involvement in Patient Safety: What Factors Influence Patient Participation and Engagement? Health Expect 2007; 10(3):259-67.
35. ECC Committee, Subcommittees and Task Forces of the American Heart Association. 2005 American Heart Association Guidelines for Cardiopulmonary Resuscitation and Emergency Cardiovascular Care. Circulation 2005; 112(24 Suppl): IV1-203.
36. Edwards S. Nursing Ethics: A Principle-Based Approach. Macmillan, Basingstoke: 2009.
37. Resuscitation Council (UK). Decisions Relating to Cardiopulmonary Resuscitation: A Joint Statement from the British Medical Association, the Resuscitation Council (UK) and the Royal College of Nursing. RC (UK), London. https://www.resus.org.uk/dnacpr/decisions-relating-to-cpr/ Accessed on 13 January 2015.
38. Agard A, Hermeren G, Herlitz J. Should Cardiopulmonary Resuscitation be Performed on Patients with Heart Failure? The Role of the Patient in the Decision-Making Process. J Intern Med 2000; 248(4):279-86.
39. Brett B, Peak EJ, Nair A, et al. Do Not Resuscitate Decisions. More Consumer Education and Involvement are Needed. BMJ 2001; 322(7278):103-4.
40. Luce JM. Physicians Do Not Have a Responsibility to Provide Futile or Unreasonable Care if a Patient or Family Insists. Crit Care Med 1995; 23(4):760-6.
41. Baskett P, Steen P, Bossaert L. The Ethics of Resuscitation and End of Life Decisions. In Baskett P, Nolan J (Eds). A Pocket Book of the European Resuscitation Council Guidelines for Resuscitation 2005. Mosby Elsevier, Edinburgh: 194-210.
42. British Medical Association (BMA), Resuscitation Council (UK) Royal College of Nursing. Decisions Relating to Cardiopulmonary Resuscitation: A Joint Statement. J Med Ethics 2001; 27:310-316.
43. Hilberman M, Kutner J, Parsons D, et al. Marginally Effective Medical Care: Ethical Analysis of Issues in Cardiopulmonary Resuscitation (CPR). J Med Ethics 1997; 23(6):361-7.
44. Willard C. Cardiopulmonary Resuscitation for Palliative Care Patients: A Discussion of Ethical Issues. Palliat Med 2000; 14(4):308-12.

45. Thompson IE, Melia KM, Boyd KM, et al, eds. Nursing Ethics. 5th ed. Edinburgh: Churchill Livingstone, 2006.
46. Hutchinson C. Addressing Issues Related to Adult Patients Who Lack the Capacity to Give Consent. Nurs Stand 2005; 19(23):47-53.
47. UK Clinical Ethics Network. The Four Principles of Biomedical Ethics. http://www.ukcen.net/index.php/ethical_issues/ethical_frameworks/the_four_princi ples_of_biomedical_ethics Accessed on 25 June 2007.
48. Noble-Adams R. Ethics and Nursing Research 1: Development, Theories and Principles. Br J Nurs 1999; 8(13):888-92.
49. Ebrahim AM. Euthanasia (qatl al-rahma). J Islam Med Assoc 2007; 39:173-8.
50. Sarhill N, LeGrand S, Islambouli R, et al. The Terminally Ill Muslim: Death and Dying from the Muslim Perspective. Am J Hosp Palliat Care 2001; 18(4):251-5.
51. Portal of the General Presidency of Scholarly Research and Ifta. Fatwa No. 12086 (Hijra). http://www.alifta.net/Fatawa/fatawaDetails.aspx?languagename=en&BookID=7&View=Page&PageNo=1&PageID=9767 Accessed on 13 January 2015.
52. IMANA Ethics Committee. Islamic Medical Ethics: the IMANA perspective. J Islam Med Assoc 2005; 37:33-42.
53. IMANA Ethics Committee. Islamic Medical Association of North America. Death. J Islam Med Assoc 1997; 29:99.
54. Takrouri MSM, Halwani TM. An Islamic Medical and Legal Prospective of Do Not Resuscitate Order in Critical Care Medicine. The Internet Journal of Health 2007; 7. http://ispub.com/IJH/7/1/10044 Accessed 10 December 2009.
55. LaFollette H. Ethics in Practice: An Anthology. Oxford: Wiley-Blackwell, 2014: 25–26.
56. Curlin FA. Euthanasia in Severely Ill Newborns. N Engl J Med 2005; 352(22):2353-5.
57. Encyclopedia Britannica. Hippocratic Oath. http://www.britannica.com/topic/Hippocratic-oath Accessed on 13 January 2015.
58. Translation of Sahih Bukhari, Book 71. University of Southern California. Hadith 7.71.670. http://www.quranexplorer.com/Hadith/English/Hadith/bukhari/007.071.670.html Accessed on 17 March 2016.

59. Translation of Sahih Muslim, Book 35. University of Southern California. Hadith 35.6485.http://www.usc.edu/org/cmje/religious-texts/hadith/muslim/035-mt.php Accessed on 17 March 2016.
60. Translation of Sahih Muslim. Book 35. University of Southern California. Hadith 35.6480. http://www.usc.edu/org/cmje/religious-texts/hadith/muslim/035-smt.php Accessed on 17 March 2016.
61. Sacred Congregation for the Doctrine of the Faith. Declaration on Euthanasia. http://www.vatican.va/roman_curia/congregations/cfaith/documents/rc_con_cfaith_ doc_19800505_euthanasia_en.html Accessed on 13 January 2015.

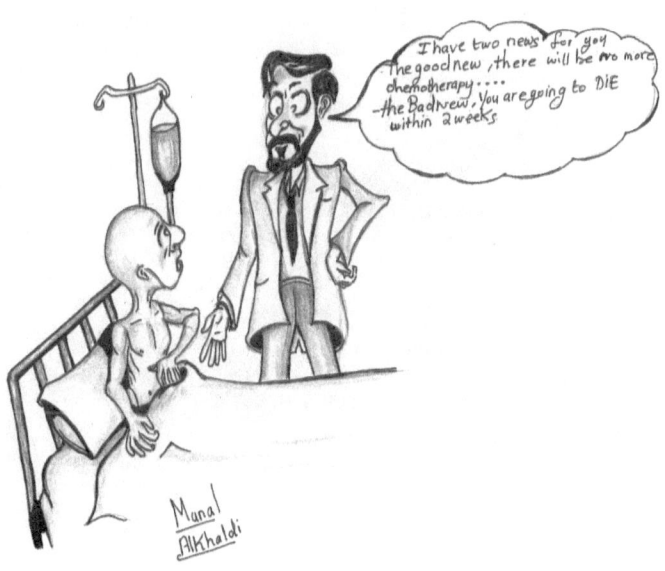

ETHICS OF GASTROINTESTINAL ENDOSCOPY

Omar Sharif

The explosive development of gastroenterology and gastrointestinal endoscopy with the new development of sophisticated endoscopes and endoscopic accessories led to an increase in diagnostic and therapeutic endoscopic procedures[1]. In the past decades, patient relied completely on the integrity of the doctor concerned to decide the benefit of the diagnostic or therapeutic intervention needed because the "doctor is always right"[2].

Currently, the number of elderly patients in our society has increased, and palliative endoscopic procedures and interventions have become common with the success of medicine to prolong life. Informed consent in the elderly and decision-making about intervention has become an issue of concern. All these concerns raise some ethical issues that have become a daily question in the endoscopy suite.

The development of new endoscopic techniques that aid into the insertion of gastric feeding tubes unlocks the subject of feeding in elderly and the impact on their lives.

A patient coming to the endoscopy suite expects a painless procedure and patient satisfaction has become a major issue in the medical practice.

Endoscopic screening for malignant and premalignant lesions in the gastrointestinal tract has become a major role of the gastroenterologist. The development of organized screening programs in the western countries and the positive result of the reduction of mortality and morbidity from colon cancer has made screening in the Middle East a necessity. Changing the mindset of the patient to undergo an invasive procedure while he has no symptoms is a major challenge to the gastroenterologist, especially considering social issues and patient education.

In this chapter, the author will try to discuss the subject mentioned above and the ethical issues that evolve.

Informed Consent

Over the last 50 years, informed consent has undergone a transformation from an ethical concept to a legal doctrine. It is based on the ethical principles of self-determination and autonomy[3]. For any proposed procedure or treatment, the physicians have the primary responsibility to disclose to patients the diagnosis, nature, risks and benefits, and reasonably available alternatives before obtaining the consent[4].

In our society, the principle of decision-making by the patient rather than the physician is yet to develop. There is still a complete reliance on the doctor's decision. These concepts do improve with the increase in the educational level of the patient. That puts an extra responsibility on the doctor to explain the procedure well and justify every intervention made.

Another issue of the informed consent is the fact that some of the patients, especially in our society, do not want to know the nature of the procedure, the diagnosis "especially when it is about malignancy", and they do not want to know the nature of any potential complications that could occur with endoscopy. That puts the physician between the ethical obligation of disclosure of information to the patient and the social pressure of hiding or "sugar-coating" the potential outcomes and the diagnosis.

Informed consent is an essential legal document. Patient understanding of the outcomes of endoscopy and potential complication would lower the possibility of legal persecution if any of those complications were to occur.

Definition of Informed Consent

"Informed consent is defined as a physician's legal requirement to disclose information to his or her patient and enables the patient to understand, evaluate, and authorize a specific surgical or medical intervention[5]".

There are two standards of disclosure. The "Physician-based standard" implies that the doctor would disclose information that another physician would understand. The "Patient-based standard", in which, the doctor must provide information that a reasonable layperson would consider substantial and significant[6]. I believe the "Patient-based" standard is more reasonable especially in our part of the world.

Information to Be Disclosed

The essential elements of disclosure include the following:

1. The patient's pertinent medical diagnosis and test results.
2. The nature of the proposed procedure.
3. The reason the procedure is being suggested.
4. The benefits of the procedure.
5. The risks and complications of the procedure, including the relative incidence and severity that would be significant to the patient's decision-making process.

6. Reasonable alternatives to the proposed procedure.
7. The patient's prognosis if the treatment or test is declined[7].

Significant risks that would influence a reasonable person to make a choice are required including the probability and severity of possible outcomes, not all possible risks/complications to be disclosed.

Who Should Obtain the Informed Consent?

The endoscopist is the best person to obtain the consent, and it is advised that she/he should do it in most cases. If not, a senior doctor who is involved in the care of the patient and can explain the risks and benefits should be the one obtaining the consent. In some hospitals, a nurse would obtain the consent, which would be accepted if the nurse is competent enough to explain the procedure. The legal liability of a nurse obtaining the consent might differ in different countries.

A questionnaire study showed that trainees involved in surgical procedures were often not able to correctly enumerate all the risks, benefits and alternatives procedures of informed consent[8].

The ethical obligation makes the primary endoscopist the sole responsible individual, making sure that the patient or his caregiver is aware and that the consent process was done effectively.

Who Is Eligible to Provide Informed Consent

The informed consent should be obtained from the patient unless the patient is a minor or deemed mentally incompetent to give informed consent. In that case, a legal guardian should provide the consent. In the case of a mentally incompetent patient, the next of kin or an individual with legal power of attorney should provide the consent. It is ethically and legally not accepted to obtain consent from a distant relative or a friend unless there was no other alternative, and in these cases, the doctor could make a medical decision especially if the procedure is considered an emergency.

The practice of obtaining consent from a relative without talking to the patient himself even when he is competent is quite common in our part of the world. It is commonly justified by some people to avoid disclosing a life-threatening diagnosis or to "sugar coat" a complication of a procedure to the patient. That raises a major ethical issue, but social barriers are sometimes hard to break in these circumstances.

Withholding information from patients at their request is a legally recognized exception to informed consent and is referred to as a waiver[6]. A patient may elect to waive the right to informed consent.

When there is inadequate time because of clinical emergency and there is a threat to a patient's life, the treating endoscopist may forgo informed consent and proceed with the procedure.

Documentation of Informed Consent

Most hospitals require written documentation of the consent (consent form) to satisfy their informed consent policies. Policies are essential for legal and ethical reasons.

The specific details and complications concerning different procedures should be documented (ERCP or PEG tube placement).

Consent for Screening Procedures

Informed consent for screening endoscopy is important because of the elective nature of the procedure. Iatrogenic complication assumes greater ethical significance and suggests that the patient should understand not only the processes of the procedure, but also its purpose and alternatives. The iatrogenic injury may include false-positive findings with needless additional testing or from false-negative with missed lesions, as well as the direct complications of the procedure[9].

Patient Satisfaction and Sedation in Endoscopy

Patient satisfaction is an important issue in achieving excellence in health care. Satisfaction in Endoscopy has its own complexities.

Multiple factors can affect satisfaction in endoscopy including[10]:

1. The technical quality of care, including the skills of the endoscopist
2. The comfort and tolerability of the procedure
3. The "art" of care (the personal manner of the endoscopy staff)
4. The provision of an adequate explanation of the procedure
5. Communication with the physicians before and after the procedure
6. The endoscopy suite environment
7. Waiting time or delays

In the United States, most endoscopies are performed with conscious sedation. In Europe and Middle East, sedation is used less frequently, and it has been expected by most patients that sedation will not be complete during endoscopy.

Multiple factors affect patient's tolerance to endoscopy. Male patients and those above the age of 50 are more tolerant to endoscopy compared to those with prior experience to endoscopy[11]. Females, patients below 50, people with pharyngeal hypersensitivity and those undergoing endoscopy for the first time experience more anxiety and are less tolerant to the procedure.

In a study reported by Abrahams et al, only 61% of patients rated the comfort of the procedure without sedation as "acceptable"[11]. Therefore, sedation is a major part of patient's satisfaction and sometimes performing the procedure without sedation would lead to complications.

Sedation should be offered to patient undergoing endoscopy and in anxious patients.

Midazolam, Diazepam, Pethidine and Fentanyl are safe, but require monitoring of oxygen saturation and pulse rate. On the other hand, Propofol induces deep sedation, and this is a major advantage for painless colonoscopy in selected patients.

Over-sedation can induce respiratory depression and recovery delay in elderly patients and patients with cardiopulmonary risk factors.

Patient privacy is a crucial issue during sedation. Ensuring the privacy of the patient is important, particularly a female with the presence of male endoscopist and endoscopy nurses and staff. A chaperone of the same gender of the patient should be present, and the patient's preference should be discussed.

Patient's satisfaction should be assessed after the procedure to improve the services in the endoscopy unit. Satisfaction could be achieved via a personal interview, a written questionnaire or email.

Endoscopy in the Elderly

Our population is aging, and the number of elderly patients requiring endoscopy has increased. Ethical issues should be considered in the elderly, especially limited life expectancy and the complexity of health problems and difficulties in obtaining informed consent. It might be appropriate to continue screening for colorectal neoplasia in the elderly as long as there are no life-limiting co-morbidities.

Informed Consent in the Elderly

Informed consent should be obtained from the patient as long as he is mentally competent to make a decision. The cognitive function of the elderly patient should be assessed and other physical limitations (vision and hearing) should be considered.

If the consent is to be obtained from the patient, it should be done preferably in the presence of the family and the information should be provided earlier for consideration[12].

If the patient is deemed incompetent to make a decision, the next of kin or a legal guardian should give the consent. In the Arab world, families can be large and multiple family members would want to be involved in the decision-making about endoscopy and other medical decisions. It is very important ethically and legally that the family should delegate a representative who should be the primary decision-maker in these situations.

Sedation in the Elderly

Sedation comes with its risk. Cardiovascular disease and pulmonary dysfunction are limitations that should be considered in every patient. Elderly patients come with more comorbid conditions that would make sedation a higher risk. Elderly patients are more susceptible to sedation complications and overdose compared to younger patients.

Data shows that elderly patients tolerate not sedated diagnostic endoscopy more than younger patients[13,14].

When offering endoscopy to the elderly, sedation risks and alternatives should be discussed and documented in the informed consent. Minimal sedation in lower doses can be offered safely to the elderly while providing comfort and diligent monitoring.

Screening for Premalignant Lesions in the Elderly

Colon cancer screening and screening for Barrett's esophagus are part of the gastroenterologist's daily work, but in the elderly, it should be considered "is screening necessary?" "The United States Preventive Services Task Force (USPSTF) guidelines recommend that patients over age 85 are not to be screened, and recommend against screening in adults 76 to 85 years unless there is an individual consideration that favors screening[15]".

Patient life expectancy and comorbid conditions should be considered. A logical and ethical question should be contemplated: "What if we find cancer?", "Are we going to proceed to surgery or the procedure would be at a higher risk?" Patient wishes should be considered in all these cases.

Palliative Endoscopy

Palliative endoscopy for terminal malignancy represents a small part of the wide spectrum of interventions, including drug therapies, psychological, religious and social aids to maintain the quality of life[1].

Biliopancreatic, esophageal obstruction, small bowel and colon obstruction have potential therapeutic endoscopic possibility to alleviate pain, provide comfort for terminal illness and provide enteral nutrition such as esophageal stenting in esophageal cancer. Celiac plexus anesthesia can be accomplished endoscopically and can lead to excellent control of pain that can be sustained for a patient with abdominal malignancy.

It is possible to help patients to live with their serious terminal illness, but a physician should not have the illusion of making human live beyond the inherent life-span[16].

The major ethical question is "when to stop therapy". Decision makers should keep in mind that those endoscopic interventions are aimed at comfort and not cure. Certain manifestations, such as anorexia, fatigue and depression are sometimes difficult to alleviate. Life expectancy, anatomical limits, risks and cost should all be considered.

A very important issue is honesty about the prognosis; it is essential to explain the situation to the patient and his family and avoid giving false expectations.

Ethical Issues of Percutaneous Endoscopic Gastrostomy Tube Placement and Artificial Nutrition

Percutaneous Endoscopic Gastrostomy (PEG) placement is an endoscopic procedure developed in the early 1980s; an endoscopist places a tube in the stomach without the need for surgery.

PEG replaced surgical gastrostomy. It replaced the need for prolonged nasogastric tube placement which could lead, after a prolonged period, to complications, such as severe ulceration in the nasal mucosa, pharynx and esophagus, severe infections and sinusitis. In addition to other discomforts, cosmetic and emotional effect to families seeing their loved one with a tube protruding from the nose should be considered.

If artificial nutrition is needed, a PEG tube should be placed and not a long-term nasogastric tube.

The issues of artificial nutrition and hydration and placement of PEG are a challenging medical/ethical issues. It is ethically and legally accepted that artificial nutrition is a medical treatment.

Many patients and their families view artificial nutrition and hydration as basic healthcare that should never be denied to any patient. This myth continues to be held by healthcare providers who may feel obligated to offer some form of treatment to a patient who is otherwise dying[16].

There is an emotional aspect in placing a PEG tube because physicians sometimes feel that withholding feeding is similar to "starving" the patient to death.

The decision to place a PEG tube should be considered based on the benefits of the procedure to the patient.

Medical indications of placing a PEG tube:

- Esophageal obstruction
- Dysphagia without obstruction
- Refusal to swallow without evidence of concomitant terminal illness
- Supplemental nutrition for patients undergoing chemo/radiation therapy with or without surgery with impaired nutrition
- Chronic gastric decompression in patients with benign/malignant obstruction who do not wish or cannot have a nasogastric tube

Some indications for placing a PEG tube have a debatable benefit, such as in vegetative state and the demented, geriatric patients.

In a vegetative state, discussion about long-term care should be discussed with the family. If life-prolonging measures are to be taken, placement of a PEG tube is indicated. There might be no physiological benefit to placing it, but no feeding will lead to physiological derangement that would lead to patient demise. Therefore, the decision of PEG tube placement should be discussed along with ventilator support, inotropic dialysis therapy and other life-prolonging measures.

In the case of the demented elderly, the issue is more complicated and controversial. Many of these elderly have Alzheimer's disease or multiple infarcts; it is unfortunate that some expect that enteral nutrition will provide comfort to the dying elderly[16].

In many cases, oral nutrition could be provided. Review of medications and avoiding anticholinergic, benzodiazepines and neuroleptics could lead to an improvement of the mental status and eventually improve oral nutrition.

Many studies revealed no clinical benefits from PEG tube placement and artificial nutrition and hydration in the demented population and advised against the procedure in such group[18,19]. Furthermore, many of these studies did not show physiological benefits[17]. Other studies reported life prolongation and better care with the placement of PEG tube[17,20,21].

PEG tube should be placed when there is a clear indication. In the demented elderly and patient in vegetative state, discussion with the family should be initiated. The issue is still controversial and could be ethical. A nasogastric tube should not be a replacement for PEG tube for long-term feeding.

Malpractice in Endoscopy

Endoscopy is an invasive procedure which could lead to several serious complications.

The endoscopist is liable only for the adverse effects due to negligence. An adverse outcome due to the illness and a perforation resulting from a properly indicated colonoscopy for which informed consent was correctly obtained is not the responsibility of the endoscopist[2].

Common Causes of Malpractice in Endoscopy

- ➤ Suboptimal performance
- ➤ Iatrogenic injuries: perforation or post-ERCP pancreatitis. These could be expected complications and should be mentioned in every informed consent

- ➤ Medication errors: sedation or medications prescribed after endoscopy
- ➤ Diagnostic errors: the most common being missed polyps or cancers on screening colonoscopy
- ➤ Informed consent: the main issues in most malpractice cases. It is very important to be performed accurately, documented well, and the expected complications explained

In many countries in the Middle East, malpractice laws are not very clear. There is less likelihood of legal action to be taken against physicians' malpractice. Therefore, the endoscopist's ethics should be the mainstay to protect the patients. More strict malpractice laws should be applied to protect patients and doctors as well.

Screening Colonoscopy in the Middle East

Colon cancer is a major cause of death and morbidity worldwide. Colon cancer screening prevents or reduces morbidity and mortality by either finding cancer early or removing precancerous polyps. Colonoscopy has become the standard of care in colon cancer screening in Europe and North America.

The reluctance to undergo an invasive procedure, such as endoscopy without symptoms has always been a problem. In the west, that was overcome by extensive educational programs.

In our part of the world, colonoscopy is difficult to perform since it involves sensitive personal parts of the body and the high level of reluctance to medical care in general unless someone is truly sick. Other alternatives to screening colonoscopy are available, but not so effective.

The endoscopist is a professional, and his/her ethical duty is to educate and consider the social aspects of colonoscopy, but at the same time not go with the flow of social resistance.

CONCLUSION

The complications of this elective procedure should be explained in detail and not to be underestimated. An important issue is the risk of missed lesions; therefore, the endoscopist should not give a false impression to the patient that the procedure will protect him/her completely from getting cancer.

Another issue in screening colonoscopy is what age it should not be offered. In our society, we tend to ignore screening procedures in a younger age compared to Western societies. As doctors, we should keep the same standards of care, putting into consideration the social aspects, patient comorbidities and the available resources.

REFERENCES

1. Ladas SD, Novis B, Triantafyllou K, et al. Ethical Issues in Endoscopy: Patient Satisfaction, Safety in Elderly Patients, Palliation, and Relations with Industry. Second European Symposium on Ethics in Gastroenterology and Digestive Endoscopy, Kos, Greece, July 2006. Endoscopy 2007; 39(6):556-65.
2. Stanciu C, Ladas S. Medical Ethics, Focus of Diagnostic and Therapeutic Endoscopy 2002, 96-112.
3. Making Health Care Decisions. The Ethical and Legal Implications of Informed Consent in the Patient-Practitioner Relationship. Available at: http://kie.georgetown.edu/nrcbl/documents/pcemr/makingdecisions.pdf.
4. LeBlang TR. Informed Consent and Disclosure in the Physician-Patient Relationship: Expanding Obligations for Physicians in the United States. Med Law 1995; 14(5-6):429-44.
5. Pape T. Legal and Ethical Considerations of Informed Consent. AORN J 1997; 65(6):1122-7.
6. ASGE. Informed Consent for GI Endoscopy. Available at: http://www.asge.org/assets/0/71542/71544/279c89a3-4acf-46e1-aaed-24c2b37e70df.pdf.

7. Barry R, Furrow TL, Greaney SH, et al. Health law. 2nd ed. St. Paul (Minn): West Group; 2000: 311-343.
8. Angelos P, DaRosa DA, Bentram D, et al. Residents Seeking Informed Consent: are They Adequately Knowledgeable? Curr Surg 2002; 59(1):115-8.
9. Thorevska N, Tilluckdharry L, Ticko S, et al. Informed Consent for Invasive Medical Procedures from the Patient's Perspective. Conn Med 2004; 68(2):101-5.
10. Yacavone RF, Locke GR 3rd, Gostout CJ, et al. Factors Influencing Patient Satisfaction with GI Endoscopy. Gastrointest Endosc 2001; 53(7):703-10.
11. Abraham NS, Wieczorek P, Huang J, et al. Assessing Clinical Generalizability in Sedation Studies of Upper GI Endoscopy. Gastrointest Endosc 2004; 60(1):28-33.
12. Ladas SD. Informed Consent: Still Far from Ideal. Digestion 2006; 73: 187-8.
13. Abraham NS, Fallone CA, Mayrand S, et al. Sedation versus No Sedation in the Performance of Diagnostic Upper Gastrointestinal Endoscopy: A Canadian Randomized Controlled Cost-Outcome Study. Am J Gastroenterol 2004; 99(9):1692-9.
14. Takahashi Y, Tanaka H, Kinjo M, et al. Sedation-Free Colonoscopy. Dis Colon Rectum 2005; 48(4):855-9.
15. Lieberman DA, Weiss DG, Bond JH, et al. Use of Colonoscopy to Screen Asymptomatic Adults for Colorectal Cancer. Veterans Affairs Cooperative Study Group 380. N Engl J Med 2000; 343(3):162-8.
16. Angus F, Burakoff R. The Percutaneous Endoscopic Gastrostomy Tube. Medical and Ethical Issues in Placement. Am J Gastroenterol 2003; 98(2):272-7.
17. Glick SM, Jotkowitz AB. Feeding Dementia Patients via Percutaneous Endoscopic Gastrostomy. Annals Long-Term Care 2013; 21(1).
18. Mendiratta P, Tilford JM, Prodhan P, et al. Trends in Percutaneous Endoscopic Gastrostomy Placement in the Elderly from 1993 to 2003. Am J Alzheimers Dis Other Demen 2012; 27(8):609-13.
19. Finucane TE, Christmas C, Travis K. Tube Feeding in Patients with Advanced Dementia: A Review of the Evidence. JAMA 1999; 282(14):1365-70.

20. Clarfield AM, Monette J, Bergman H, et al. Enteral Feeding in End-Stage Dementia: A Comparison of Religious, Ethnic, and National Differences in Canada and Israel. J Gerontol A Biol Sci Med Sci 2006; 61(6):621-7.
21. Norberg A, Hirschfeld M, Davidson B, et al. Ethical Reasoning Concerning the Feeding of Severely Demented Patients: an International Perspective. Nurs Ethics. 1994; 1(1):3-13.

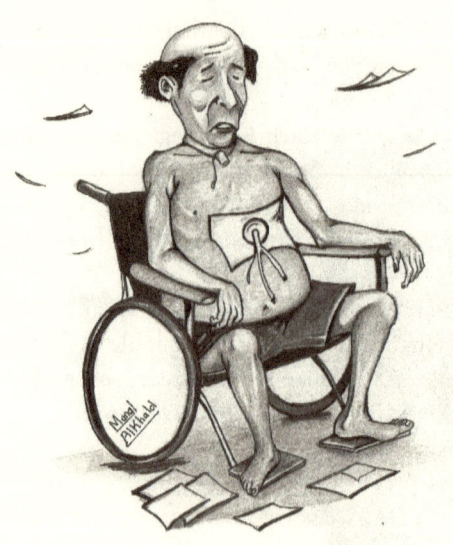

ETHICS IN NURSING AND THE NURSING PROCESS

Fairouz Alhourani, Sharon Skowronski

Nursing as a career in the Middle East was undesirable, and this had an adverse effect on recruitment, which led to a shortage of nurses. In Bahrain, the nursing profession was considered an unsuitable career for their daughters, largely due to the perception of low status, unsocial working hours, low income and other cultural reasons[1]. Therefore, there had been a reliance on recruiting nurses from overseas, including the Philippines, India, South Africa, United Kingdom and other Middle Eastern countries to cover the shortfall.

Since the 1960s, Bahrain healthcare service has continued to expand, which increased the need for more nurses to be trained within Bahrain to fulfill identified shortages and eventually reduce the need for overseas nurses.

Because of the introduction of level degree programs and the understanding of the local health service to improve working conditions, the interest for local Bahraini females to make a career in nursing has increased. It was suggested that the attitude towards nursing in the Arab world has improved in recent years[2]. Consequently, there has been a recognition of the need for regulations and licensing for nurses. That led to the publication of "The Regulation of Practicing Nursing and Midwifery" in 1987[3].

In 1991, Bahrain Nursing Service was established to further develop the nursing profession and the Bahrain National Code of Professional Conduct for Nurses was published in 2002, an interpretation of the Gulf Cooperation Council (GCC) Professional Code of Practice for Nurses.

The aim of the code is to give guidance for a conduct consistent with the ethical obligations of the nursing profession, to deliver a high standard of nursing care, to provide a framework for ethical decisions and to enable the nurse to exercise professional self-regulation[4].

Professional codes of conduct for nurses in individual countries followed the introduction of the International Code of Ethics (1953) which was revised in 2012 by the International Council of Nurses. Fundamentally, the codes set out four responsibilities for nurses: to promote health, prevent illness, restore health and alleviate suffering[5].

Nurses have an obligation to practice in a manner that is lawful and accepted by the countries' code of practice[6]. However, in practice, the law does not always provide the answers to how a nurse deals with complex situations or dilemmas, for example, in the scenario of the dying patient. A doctor may decide that a patient with a painful terminal illness should not be resuscitated. He may consider that what he is suggesting is ethically right and in the best interest of the patient. But the nurse may feel that due to her cultural beliefs and upbringing, the patient's life should be sustained at all cost. In this scenario, both of these professionals would not be intending to act unlawfully, but their decision would be considered as a morality issue[7].

Thompson et al suggested that morals and ethics are terms used to refer to social customs regarding what is wrong and right in practice and theory of human behavior. Moreover, moral is what the person believes is wrong or right based on their culture, upbringing, education and religion[8].

According to Lewis et al, ethics is a system of moral principles. They underpin how an individual and society live their lives and make their decisions[9]. Therefore, this chapter is aimed at broadening the understanding of the spectrum of ethics, in the context of nurses, how they are constantly being challenged with ethical dilemmas within their practice. The nursing process will also be discussed to highlight the interplay between the different ethical theories that underpin the nurse's actions and therapeutic relationship with the patient.

Objective of Ethics

The scope of ethics includes the individual's morals and values during the promotion of the greater good for people. That may involve common dilemmas such as abortion, human rights and professional conduct. The objective of ethical theories is to guide human behavior. Thus, ethics is used as a guide with the nurse making the eventual decision[10].

Ethics and People

Ethics could be a source of group strength, and as such, it may at times be used as a weapon. At times, ethics can be used as ammunition to target other people who appear immoral[10].

Nursing Ethics and Medical Ethics are based on similar principles of beneficence, non-maleficence, respect and autonomy; however, Nursing Ethics focuses more on human relationship and collaborative care[11].

Brief History of Ethics in Nursing

Professional nurses were once trained by male physicians. Subsequently, this led to nurses focusing on the technical aspects of nursing as opposed to the human relation which Nightingale advocated[12]. In 1899, the International Council of Nurses (ICN) launched the first Code of Ethics. That was followed by the first nursing ethical book authored by Isabel Hampton Robb in 1990. However, her work seemed to describe the "obedient" nurse as a physician's "handmaiden" and included chapter writings based on Uniform, Night-Duty, and Care of the Patient, and nurse-physician, nurse-nurse, nurse-public relationships. This submissive notion appeared to continue till 1965 as a reflection of the ICN Code of Ethics.

In 1973, the nursing responsibility shifted towards the patient and away from a physician's "hand-maiden"[12].

Nursing Ethics underscore what it is to care for a patient, as opposed to "curing" a patient.

Nursing Ethics is the caring and the holistic focus of the patient as "human" and not a disease or illness[13].

Ethical Dilemmas and Challenges in Nursing

Nurses often face ethical dilemmas in their practice. Despite the presence of guidelines that are morally acceptable. It may be inevitable that there are still issues, which could be considered gray.

According to Butts et al, no code could provide absolute or complete rules that are free of conflict and ambiguity. True enough, even the different ethical theories vary on their stand and may point to different decisions based on similar situations[12].

Because of the different perspective on ethics, nurses are facing challenges/problems, often without satisfactory resolution[12].

Common Ethical Dilemmas and Challenges in Nursing

Freedom versus Control

Sometimes, the duty to benefit the patient (beneficence) and avoiding harm (non-maleficence) will come into direct conflict with other ethical principles such as respecting the patient's autonomy[14]. More often, nurses are in a dilemma whether to ensure patient autonomy or to be much more paternalistic in his/her approach, especially if patient's actions might be detrimental to his/her health.

Nurses might ask, "Does the patient have the right to make choices for one's self that may result in harm or should the nurse prevent this choice?"

Example: If a patient decides to be discharged against medical advice and does not want his/her family to know about it. The nurse knows that the action is detrimental to the patient's health since treatments would be discontinued. The nurse would be in a dilemma whether to honor the patient's autonomy or to act on behalf of the patient and inform the family so the family may avert the patient's decision.

Benefitting the Patient

The nurse's core of caring is the patient. However, problems arise because nurses have the difficulty to determine which action is beneficial to the patient. Will the nurse focus on producing the greatest possible general health benefit for the patient or emphasize only on the specific benefit for the disease condition?

Furthermore, which one should be given priority, to benefit the patient or to avoid harm? A nurse might also ask whether to do what is beneficial in individual cases or to think in broader terms, such as what is beneficial to many?[14].

Justice: The Allocation of Scarce Resources

Allocating the nursing time might be difficult, some nurses might be confronted with the dilemma of who should be apportioned most of the time. For example, trained nurses in critically ill patients unit where the number of patients exceeds the number of nurses: how does one determine which patients deserve to be cared for by a critically-care trained nurse?[14] Some nurses might consider the principle of beneficence while others calculate the benefits and the harms.

Respect: How Can It Be Shown to Patients?

Respect in nursing practice is to make patient needs a priority and provide care in a dignified manner.

However, one issue that nurses face: how "persons" is defined. Many secular refers to a "person" as someone who is self-aware or self-conscious[14]. By that definition, fetuses, or living individuals who are not orientated and are unconscious, (such as with a Glasgow Coma Score of 3) may not be considered as "persons."

Veracity versus Deception

It is imperative that the truth is disclosed. Telling the truth is believed to be morally acceptable. However, there are often situations where nurses are confronted with challenges regarding veracity. Perhaps nurses are bound to the idea of "benevolent deceptions" wherein patients are not told the truth to protect patients from the ill-effects of bad news[14].

Nonetheless, there is doubt if the good motive underlying withholding information from the patient justifies deception. Some philosophers, however, would say that the patients have the right to know the truth regardless of the consequences.

"What if deception would benefit the patient?" "How sure are we that withholding the truth would benefit the patient?" "Would the benefit of withholding the information outweigh the harms of telling the truth?"

Fidelity: Is it Morally Acceptable to Break a Promise?

Most nurses recognize that there is a moral obligation to respect and keep commitments. That is known as fidelity or promise keeping. Nurses might ask whether, in certain situations, it is morally acceptable to break the promise. Again, nurses would be looking at the consequences, the benefits and the harms.

Another aspect of fidelity is keeping patient's confidence, better known as keeping confidentiality. There is a great debate as to what are the situations that will allow nurses to break a patient's confidence. Fry et al maintain that the moral basis of confidentiality remains unclear[14].

The Sanctity of Human Life

It could not be denied that many people from different cultural or religious backgrounds view human life as sacred. It cannot be avoided that the idea of the sanctity of human life gives rise to many issues, controversies and dilemma in nursing ethics[14].

Often, such issues revolve around patients who are inevitably dying. Nurses are often trapped in situations where they have to choose between action and omission. Some morally challenging questions may include: "Is it morally preferable to withhold treatment and let nature takes its course by allowing natural death than to intervene actively to kill the patient?" "Is withdrawing a treatment that has already been started in dying patients considered actively participating in the patient's death?"

Another dilemma that nurses face includes Advance Directives. Nurses are torn between absolutely following patient's advance directives of not starting treatment despite the fact that treatment has a great benefit for the patient.

There are also controversies revolving around the administration of medications which alleviate the pain of a dying patient, but at the same time have certain side effects that may hasten a patient's death, such as if a nurse is asked to administer a high dosage of Morphine to a patient with a terminal stage of lung cancer. The nurse knows the effects of high dose of Morphine and might be in a dilemma of whether to give the medication or not. Ethical decision-making could be very difficult because of different ethical issues. That might result in a significant physical and emotional stress as expressed by the American Association of Critical-Care Nurses (AACN)[15].

Moral distress contributes to the feeling of loss of integrity and dissatisfaction with the work environment. Therefore, it is very important that nurses know how to deal with these ethical dilemmas and challenges and how to collaborate with the other healthcare team members to develop morally acceptable and ethically sound decision.

Ethics and the Nursing Process

Because of the ethical challenges that the nurses constantly face, different nursing organizations proposed their own Nursing Code of Ethics based on the International Council of Nurses (ICN) Code of Ethics[5]. The Code of Ethics refers to guidelines that shape ethical behavior and identify values and beliefs that are morally acceptable. The principle elements of the ICN Code is about nurses and people, practice, profession and co-workers.

The four elements set a standard for professionalism within nursing and reflect the ethical standards required to practice. The Nursing process is an organized approach utilized by nurses to endorse holistic patient care incorporating ethical practice[16].

Assessment is the first part of the nursing process. Assessment could be done in many ways. It may be through interviewing or physical assessment. At this stage, a collection of data about the patient, his family and/or his community is initiated[12].

During the assessment, the nurse accepts the patient's life, beliefs and values; she explores the patient's rationale for any decision despite its ill-effects. She respects the patient's choice and his wishes although she does not approve them[17]. The nurse identifies the patient's long-term and short-term goals.

The nurse plans the nursing intervention to achieve the goals identified. An individualized plan of care is formulated for the specific patient with the related nursing interventions that had been identified[12].

Confidentiality ensures that all biopsychosocial information is not shared with anyone who is not providing care or managing the patient's condition. Patients have the right to confidentiality. Relevant information may be shared with other members of the healthcare team who are also obliged to maintain patient's confidentiality. The nurse should refrain from collecting information that is unnecessary for the provision of healthcare and protecting patients' physical and emotional privacy[17].

The nurse respects the decision of the patient and explores his rationale. That portrays autonomy and respect for patient's choice. Therefore, **fidelity** is demonstrated through the nurse's actions[17].

The nurse discusses patient's diagnosis with the healthcare team and supports the patient's right to receive information, assisting the patient in understanding any information if cultural, language and literacy concerns exist. The nurse abstains from misrepresentation or deceit by giving the patient full and honest disclosure of information regarding his nursing care, displaying the ethical principle of **veracity**[17].

The nurse keeps her commitment to the patient based on her virtue of caring and her agreement to keep all promises made to the patient; therefore, advocating quality patient care. All reasonable efforts are made by the nurse to ensure patient's safety and well-being, which highlights the ethical principle of fidelity[17].

The International Code of Ethics for Nurses[10]

An international code of ethics for nurses was first adopted by the International Council of Nurses (ICN) in 1953. It has been revised and reaffirmed at various times; this review and revision were completed in 2005.

Nurses have four fundamental responsibilities: to promote health, to prevent illness, to restore health and to alleviate suffering. The need for nursing is universal.

Inherent in nursing is respect for human rights, including cultural rights, the right to life and choice, to dignity and to be treated with respect. Nursing care is respectful of and unrestricted by considerations of age, color, creed, culture, disability or illness, gender, sexual orientation, nationality, politics, race or social status.

Nurses render health services to the individual, the family, and the community and coordinate their services with those of related groups.

The ICN Code

The ICN Code of Ethics for Nurses has four principal elements that outline the standards of ethical conduct.

Elements of the Code

1. Nurses and People

The nurse's primary professional responsibility is to attend people requiring nursing care.

In providing care, the nurse promotes an environment in which the human rights, values, customs and spiritual beliefs of the individual, family and community are respected.

The nurse ensures that the individual receives sufficient information on which to base consent for care and related treatment.

The nurse holds in confidence personal information and uses judgment in sharing this information.

The nurse shares with society the responsibility for initiating and supporting action to meet the health and social needs of the public, in particular, those of vulnerable populations.

The nurse also shares the responsibility to sustain and protect the natural environment from depletion, pollution, degradation and destruction.

2. Nurses and Practice

The nurse carries personal responsibility and accountability for nursing practice and maintaining competence by continual learning.

The nurse maintains a standard of personal health such that the ability to provide care is not compromised.

The nurse uses judgment regarding individual competence when accepting and delegating responsibility.

The nurse, at all times, maintains standards of personal conduct which reflect well on the profession and enhance public confidence.

The nurse, in providing care, ensures that the use of technology and scientific advances are compatible with the safety, dignity and rights of people.

3. Nurses and the Profession

The nurse assumes the major role in determining and implementing acceptable standards of clinical nursing practice, management, research and education.

The nurse is active in developing a core of research-based professional knowledge.

The nurse, acting through the professional organization, participates in creating and maintaining safe, equitable social and economic working conditions in nursing.

4. Nurses and Co-workers

The nurse sustains a cooperative relationship with co-workers in nursing and other fields.

The nurse takes appropriate action to safeguard individuals, families and communities when their health is endangered by a co-worker or any other person.

The ICN Code of Ethics for Nurses is a guide for action based on social values and needs. It would have significance only as a living document if applied to the realities of nursing and health care in a changing society.

The four elements of the ICN Code of Ethics for Nurses: nurses and people, nurses and practice, nurses and the profession and nurses and co-workers give a framework for standards of conduct.

Nursing Practice and Codes of Conduct, Performance and Ethics

International Code of Conduct established by statutory regulatory bodies set out codes of conduct, performance and ethics for registered/licensed nursing staff. It would apply to staff in KHUH in the absence of Bahraini Legislation and code of conduct.

Codes from around the world could be summarized to contain the following principles:

The nurse in whose care the patient is placed must be trustworthy with the health and wellbeing of the patient.

To justify that trust, he/she must:

1. Make the care of people his/her priority, treating them as individuals and respecting their dignity.

2. Work with others to protect and promote the health, safety and well-being of those in his/her care, their families, carers and the wider community.
3. Provide safe, compassionate, competent and ethical care.
4. Provide a high standard of practice and care, promoting and respecting informed decision-making at all times, within their scope of practice and competence.
5. Open and honest, act with integrity and uphold the reputation of your profession.

As a professional, a nurse is personally accountable for actions and omissions in his/her practice, and must always be able to justify his/her decisions.

The Nurse Is Required to Meet the Following Standards:

1. Treat people as individuals
2. Respect people's confidentiality
3. Collaborate with those in their care
4. Ensure they gain consent
5. Share information with colleagues
6. Work effectively as part of a team
7. Delegate effectively
8. Manage risk
9. Use the best available evidence
10. Keep skills and knowledge up to date
11. Keep clear and accurate records
12. Act with integrity
13. Deal with problems
14. Be impartial
15. Be accountable
16. Engage in self-reflection and dialogue

Nurses recognize the privilege of being part of a self-regulating profession and have a responsibility to merit this privilege. The codes of conduct inform other health professionals and the public about the ethical commitments of nurses and the responsibilities nurses accept as being part of such a self-regulating profession.

CONCLUSION

Nursing ethics has come a long way since the foundations of nursing service. Though the concepts are similar to medical ethics, nursing ethics developed its identity. Rather than focusing on the cure, nursing ethics focuses on the nurturing and supportive aspects. Furthermore, ethics is intertwined throughout the nursing process, and a nurse will inevitably face ethical dilemmas. No matter what the nurse's beliefs or culture, she should always ensure that her decisions are morally sound and support the best interests of the patients and are within the Code of Ethics.

REFERENCES

1. Tawash E, Cowman S, Edgar A. A Triangulation Study: Bahraini Nursing Students' Perceptions of Nursing as a Career. Journal of Nursing Education and Practice 2012; 2(3): 81-92.
2. Shukri R. Status of Nursing in the Arab World. Ethn Dis 2005; 15(1 Suppl 1): S1-88-9.
3. Al-Naser W. The Distinguished Achievements and Pioneering Deeds of the Late Amir H.H. Shaikh Isa Bin Salman Al-Khalifa. Kingdom of Bahrain: Historical Documents Centre Publication, 1999.
4. Ministry of Health (MOH) Office of Licensure and Registration. Bahrain National Code of Professional Conduct for Nursing. The Kingdom of Bahrain, 2002.

5. International Council of Nurses. The ICN Code of Ethics for Nurses 2012. http://www.icn.ch/who-we-are/code-of-ethics-for-nurses. Accessed in 2015.
6. Nursing and Midwifery Council. Professional Standards of Practice and Behaviour for Nurses and Midwives. https://www.nmc.org.uk/globalassets/sitedocuments/nmc-publications/nmc-code.pdf Accessed in April 2015.
7. Griffith R, Tengnah C. Law and Professional Issues in Nursing. Sage Publishing, 2014: 5-38.
8. Thompson I, Melia K, Boyd K. Nursing Ethics. 4th ed. London: Churchill Livingstone, 2000.
9. Lewis MA, Tamparo CD, Tatro BM. Medical Law, Ethics and Bioethics for the Health Professions. 7th ed. Philadelphia: F.A. Davis Company, 2012.
10. British Broadcasting Corporation, 2014. Ethics Guide. http://www.bbc.co.uk/ethics/guide/ Accessed in April 2015.
11. Benner P, Tanner C, Chesla C. Expertise in Nursing Practice: Caring, Clinical Judgment and Ethics. New York: Springer Publishing Company, 2009: 171-196.
12. Butts J, Rich K. Nursing Ethics Across Curriculum and into Practice. 3rd ed. Massachusetts: Jones and Bartlett Learning, 2013: 3-85.
13. Breier-Mackie S. Medical Ethics and Nursing Ethics: Is There Really Any Difference? Gastroenterology Nursing 2006; 29(2): 182–3.
14. Fry ST, Veatch RM, Taylor CR. Case Studies in Nursing Ethics. 4th ed. Massachusetts: Jones and Bartlett Learning, 2011: 109-247.
15. American Association of Critical Care Nurses. Position Statement: Moral Distress. www.aacn.org/WD/Practice/Docs/Moral_Distress.pdf Accessed in April 2015.
16. Wingard R. Patient Education and the Nursing Process: Meeting the Patient's Needs. Nephrol Nurs J 2005; 32(2):211-4.
17. College of Nurses of Ontario. Ethics. Canada: 2009. http://www.cno.org/Global/docs/prac/41034_Ethics.pdf Accessed in April 2016.

THE ETHICS OF HYPERBARIC OXYGEN THERAPY

Adel Abdul Aal

Hyperbaric oxygen therapy is the initial medical treatment for several diseases, such as arterial gas embolism and decompression sickness. In addition, it is an adjunct treatment for clostridial myonecrosis (gas gangrene), crush injury and other acute traumatic ischemias, selected wounds, such as diabetic foot, severe anemia, necrotizing soft tissue infections, radiation tissue damage, compromised skin grafts and flaps, thermal burns and some intracranial abscesses. All these conditions are within the approved indications by the Undersea and Hyperbaric Medical Society (UHMS) and Food and Drug Administration (FDA). The FDA calls all other indications off-label[1].

Hyperbaric oxygen therapy was used in more than 130 clinical conditions and the list is increasing. Hyperbaric chambers are not only found in the hospitals and freestanding facilities, but also in private homes. Individuals also have installed chambers in homes or garages as many parents took the initiatives to treat their children. Is it ethical for a practitioner to use hyperbaric oxygen therapy for any clinical condition in which the benefit is unproven yet?[1]

The majority of hyperbaric references state that oxygen is used as a drug in the treatment of several illnesses, but it is not made by a pharmaceutical company. Therefore, this modality of treatment will not be funded for large clinical trials. Research in all areas of hyperbaric medicine has been slow. Until appropriate studies have been performed, practitioners need guidelines on how to respond to patients requesting the use of hyperbaric oxygen therapy for an off-label indication.

Is It Ethical to Use Hyperbaric Oxygen Therapy for Unproven Indications?

This question has been there since 1950s. It is not uncommon for medical practitioners to prescribe drugs and therapies from an off-label. Evidently, there is no clear guideline that allows practitioners to prescribe hyperbaric oxygen therapy for every off-label indication. It is important to draw the line for practitioners where to stop. It is essential to consider the combination of practitioner's clinical judgment, evaluation of the available scientific data and patient-informed consent[2].

Before the practitioners and patient consider an off-label indication, they must evaluate the level of scientific evidence and the risk to benefit ratio. The practitioner must understand the physiological rationale of hyperbaric oxygen therapy and whether the mechanism of action might apply to the condition of the patients. The practitioner must explain the potential benefits and risks of hyperbaric oxygen therapy for the patient. That requires the practitioner to be knowledgeable or trained in hyperbaric medicine. The patient must sign a detailed informed consent.

Informed Consent in Hyperbaric Oxygen Therapy

Practitioners must disclose the risks and benefits of hyperbaric oxygen therapy treatment, regardless of whether the indication is approved or off-label. Written informed consent should be obtained and included in the medical record of the patients. A practitioner should discuss six main issues with a patient considering off-label hyperbaric oxygen therapy as part of informed consent[2]:

1. The strength of the scientific evidence supporting the therapeutic benefits of hyperbaric oxygen therapy.
2. What are the alternative medical treatments and the cost benefits?
3. The risks of hyperbaric oxygen therapy compared to the benefits.
4. Cure or mere benefits are not guaranteed.
5. The patient should be asked to participate if a research study is available.
6. Informed consent should include disclosure of all aspects of the treatment of the patient or child's parent.

Practitioners would receive an immediate financial benefit to their unit or themselves when they administer hyperbaric oxygen therapy for an off-label indication. The practitioner is obligated to disclose any financial conflict of interest. The cost of administering the therapy should be reasonable. In the US, it is not unusual for patients to pay for off-label treatments, but it conforms to ethical standards. Patients could pay to participate in research trials if they are informed of their financial obligations and accept the fact that they are research subjects.

Research in Hyperbaric Oxygen Therapy

If hyperbaric oxygen therapy is used for an off-label indication, data should be documented for future research and analysis. Research requires approval by the Institutional Review Board (IRB) or ethical and research committee and the patients should be informed that they are research subjects[3].

Practitioners operating hyperbaric facilities or supervising patients undergoing hyperbaric oxygen treatments must be licensed and are accountable. State boards are sensitive to practitioner activities involving unproven therapies and interventions that might be considered experimental. Many freestanding facilities have no practitioner involvement, thus omitting a crucial element of supervising the progress of patients. At hospital-based facilities, practitioners who treat approved indications are expected to be physically present for the duration of the hyperbaric treatment. Maintaining compliance with the law is part of the ethical conduct of the physician[3].

CONCLUSION

Off-label and approved indication of hyperbaric oxygen therapy can be evaluated case by case, the medical condition, the patient circumstances and the available scientific data in which other medical alternatives have been explored and tried.

It is very important to all practitioners to assess the risk/benefit ratio and the cost/benefit ratio. Ethical principles should be followed: do no harm, respect for persons and beneficence. Practitioners should comply with the law, such as hyperbaric safety, promotion and advertising. The obligation of the practitioner to the patient is not merely to do what is legal, but also what is right from the standpoint of universal justice.

REFERENCES

1. Chan EC, Brody B. Ethical Dilemmas in Hyperbaric Medicine. Undersea Hyperb Med. 2001 Fall; 28(3):123-30.
2. Jacoby IJ. Hyperbaric Oxygen Therapy, Multiple Sclerosis, and Unapproved Indications: Taking a Stand. Undersea Hyperb Med. 2001 Fall; 28(3):113-5.

3. Zhai WW, Sun L, Yu ZQ, Chen G. Hyperbaric Oxygen Therapy in Experimental and Clinical Stroke. Med Gas Res. 2016 Jul 11; 6(2):111-118.

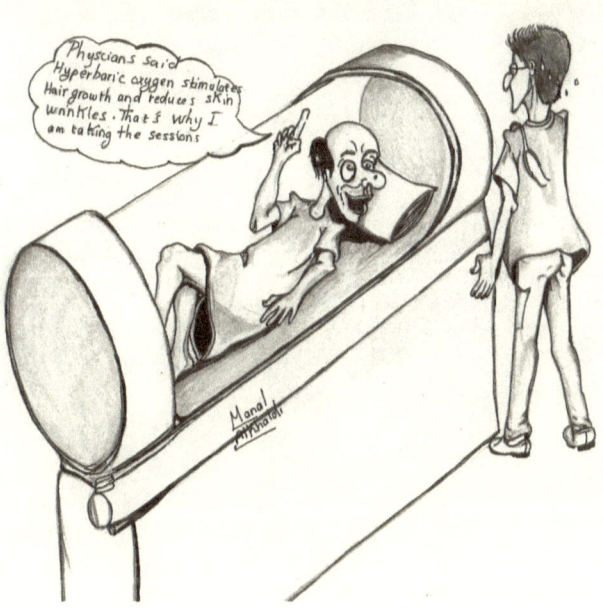

ETHICS IN THE CLINICAL LABORATORY

Suhail Baithun

Ethical behavior and moral reasoning could be a very important part of strategic decision making in healthcare. Recently, public awareness regarding ethical issues related to healthcare practice has increased including the laboratory service. These issues relate to malpractice, wasteful spending, fraud, etc.

Specific examples include providing inaccurate results to physicians and patients; thus, patients are put at risk of wrong medical management, such as the wrong blood type for transfusion or abnormal blood chemistry results.

The laboratory has a complex structure, consisting of different disciplines, including histopathology, surgical pathology, cytopathology, chemistry, hematology, blood bank, microbiology, virology, genetics and cytogenetics, toxicology and molecular biology. Laboratory staff includes medical staff (pathologists), clinical biochemists, medical laboratory technicians and phlebotomists.

It should be emphasized that all medically qualified staff take the Hippocratic Medical Oath at graduation. However, the technical staff does not take such oath. Some institutes have a similar pledge to the profession adopted by the American Society for Clinical Laboratory Science[1].

Historical Background

Medical ethics is derived from the teachings of the Greek physician, Hippocrates (460-377 BC). The ethical principles he taught still survive today as the "Hippocratic Oath". Remarkably, what he wrote 2,500 years ago is still applicable in today's practice of medicine.

ETHICS AND THE MEDICAL LABORATORY

A. General Issues

Medical laboratories are part of the medical profession and medical ethics apply to its practices.

Ethically, medical laboratories have responsibilities for the patient, the profession, colleagues and training.

1. **Duty Towards Patients**

    The laboratory's duty towards patients makes them responsible for the quality and accuracy of the laboratory services they provide, including maintaining individual competence in judgment and performance, the aim of which is safeguarding the patient. This requires laboratory staff to update their knowledge and ensure the advancement of laboratory methods and techniques.

    As professionals, laboratory staff must maintain high standards of practice; sound judgment in the assessment and performance of laboratory tests should be practiced.

    Patient information and test results must remain confidential at all times.

Confidentiality also establishes trust between the healthcare professional and the patient[4]. The principle of confidentiality emphasizes that any information related to the patient should not be divulged without his/her consent unless there are legitimate reasons supporting it[5]. According to the Code of Ethics and Professional Conducts, confidential information could be disclosed only if consented by the patient, if there is a risk to the patient or public, or if it is legally needed[6].

2. Duty to Colleagues and Profession

Laboratory staff must also have a duty to their colleagues and the profession. They must maintain the dignity and respect of the profession and aim to maintain a reputation of honesty, respect, integrity and reliability[7].

They should regularly participate in different programs to update their knowledge, such as external quality assurance programs and CMEs[8].

3. Duty to the Society

Members of the profession must contribute to the general well-being of the community[7]. A good example would be King Hamad University Hospital, which has purchased a mobile transfusion unit as an outreach to the community. That advocates members of the laboratory to go into society and have direct contact with the public.

They must comply with relevant laws and regulations related to the practice of clinical laboratory science. It must be emphasized that this should not be influenced by corporate interests driven by profit[9].

4. **Duty to Training of Junior Medical Doctors and Technical Staff**

It is part of the ethical duty of each department within the hospital to provide and create the best atmosphere for training junior medical doctors and technical staff. That must encourage junior doctors to join recognized postgraduate schemes, which offer the highest qualifications. Trainees and technical staff should be encouraged to join and attend different CME programs, conferences and performing research, audits and scientific publications. That should be part of the standards of good medical practice.

According to the GMC standards and ethical guidance for doctors, the following is included as part of Good Medical Practice: "there should be emphasis on consent, patient's confidentiality, leadership and management, raising and acting on concerns about patient safety, treatment and care towards the end of life and protecting children and young people"[10].

5. **Information Collection**

One of the most important functions of the clinical laboratory is to collect sufficient information to identify adequately patients and specimens, sufficient clinical information to perform the test accordingly and information relevant to the safety of staff and other patients.

Unfortunately, quite often, the laboratory staff deal with samples sent to the laboratory with no proper clinical information, which causes a delay in patient's management. It may take up to few days to collect the proper information. In addition, patient's identification tags must be safely attached to the container of the specimen to avoid mislabeling of the test.

Information collection needs the use of a good and reliable information technology system which should be compatible with the system of the hospital and the community[11]. This should involve information for billing purposes and resource management. As part of the openness, the patient should be aware and informed that the information has been collected and how it would be used.

6. Medical Records and the Laboratory

The laboratory must ensure that patient's records are stored with protection against loss, unauthorized access, tampering or other misuse[12].

Results must never be altered (except by properly authorized persons) in accordance with the establishment's procedures.

The department must have protocols on how long results, specimens and slides are to be kept.

7. Access to Medical Records

The information in medical records is personal and private; therefore, ethics plays an essential part in their keeping, storage and disposal[13]. The medical records are the property of the healthcare provider; however, the actual records are considered to be the property of the patient, who may obtain copies upon request.

In histopathology, requests to release patient's reports and materials for a second opinion should be authorized and consented by the patient.

8. Collection of Specimen

Informed consent should be given by mentally competent and able patients. However, in certain circumstances, consent should be given by a person responsible for the patient, such as parents/guardians or properly authorized persons.

A more detailed consent is necessary for special procedures that require invasive methods, such as a bone marrow biopsy. That would require detailed explanation to the patient of the risks and possible complications of the procedure involved.

Genetic testing would require special pre-test counseling.

It should be emphasized that any research project using patient's material should be approved by the hospital's ethical committee.

9. Performing of Tests

All tests must be carried out appropriately, which should be determined in detail by a professional organization or regulatory authorities. The laboratories must participate in different programs of internal and external quality assurance to ensure accurate results.

Each laboratory should be accredited to ensure a high level of skill and competence of the medical, scientific and allied health professions. The process of accreditation provides laboratory certification of competency and authority.

10. Results

Confidentiality is of utmost importance in laboratory practice. The result is reported to the requesting clinician.

However, results could be released to other practitioners involved with the patient's management.

The laboratory must have written standard operational procedures detailing how various requests and results should be handled and secured. That includes the responsibility for taking precautions to ensure secure and reliable methods for results delivery, which may be done through electronic means, public post or by a courier.

The prompt result is an essential part of the laboratory function to ensure swift, and proper management delivered to the patient.

As part of ethical laboratory practice, urgent critical results (blood results for myocardial infarction) should be reported immediately. Any delay in reporting these results could result in serious untoward complications including death. These results should be reported according to a KHUH bench marking[14].

An essential part of the laboratory is an accurate interpretation of results performed by qualified and accredited pathologists. Some of the results should be further discussed at different meetings, such as cancer cases at the tumor board.

11. Financial Arrangements

Financial arrangements differ from one laboratory to another. They may have their financial budget, or the budget is run by a third party, such as the hospital's Finance Department.

The laboratory has a difficult ethical responsibility if acting with limited resources, especially if provided by a third party.

B. Special Issues

1. Reproductive Technology

Assisted reproductive technology is used to treat infertility, such as in vitro fertilization, including artificial insemination, artificial reproduction, cloning, embryo transfer, fertility medication, etc.

Issues raised by discussions of reproductive technology may touch on deeply held convictions and religious beliefs[15]. The different and strongly held views on abortion, artificial insemination by donor, in vitro fertilization, intrafallopian gamete transfer and other procedures and techniques are examples of these concerns; this needs special counseling.

2. Histopathology and Cytology

The general rules for clinical pathology are applied. However, during the examination of different samples, ethical issues may be raised. For example, in the course of the examinations, certain observations may be made, such as the presence of spermatozoa on the cervical cytology smear, which is not related to the purpose of the examination. These may have social implications.

Tissue diagnosis should always provide information to assist the treating doctor. It is well-known in histopathology that the final report with the diagnosis should only be issued and signed by a consultant histopathologist.

3. Autopsy

Many religions and cultures do not accept the need for an autopsy, and this must be respected. However, an autopsy is a very important tool to reach the final diagnosis.

Every autopsy should be consented by the next of kin unless it is authorized by the coroner's office or its equivalent. The consent for autopsies is usually governed by law, and these must be followed meticulously. The consent must include sections for taking tissue for histological examination or other material, such as blood for chemistry or fluid for microbiology.

The result of the autopsy should be documented in the final report and sent to the treating doctor. Counseling the family of the deceased is recommended, where results are properly and extensively explained to the next of kin.

Tissue retention for diagnosis and research should also be properly discussed and consented.

4. **Virtual Autopsy**

Not to perform an autopsy in certain cases may raise ethical issues[16]. The chance will be lost for family counseling in cases of sudden deaths due to cardiomyopathy or cases of neonatal deaths. A virtual autopsy was recently introduced and used as an alternative to autopsy. It is a minimally-invasive imaging of the body (CT and MRI scans, withdrawals of blood or excision of tissue for toxicological assessment or histological examination) to determine the cause of death.

5. **Transfusion Medicine**

The code of ethics for blood transfusion was approved by the general assembly of the International Society of Blood Transfusion during the Society's 16th Congress held in Montreal, 1980[17].

There should be a set of standard operational procedures to protect both the blood donors and the recipients.

Donors should donate blood voluntarily without being forced and should be on a non-remunerated basis[17].

There should be standard operational procedures to ensure the protection of the donor.

The donor should be provided with adequate information about the process and should consent to donation[17].

It must be emphasized that blood should be collected under the overall supervision of a physician. In addition, confidentiality of personal details and laboratory results should be ensured.

The recipient of a blood transfusion should be provided with reliable information about the risks, benefits and any available alternatives to blood transfusion[18].

Part of the ethical issues in blood donation is the optimal use of blood products. Taking into account scarcity of blood and the dangers associated with its use; the following are misuse of blood and its products:

- Use of blood products when not clinically justified
- Use of too little or too much in patients who require transfusion
- The use of the wrong component or product for transfusion

6. HIV/AIDS

Testing for HIV/AIDS requires special consideration to protect the patient's privacy. The laboratory must ensure that samples are received with hazard signs. Patients should be fully informed of the implication if the test is positive and may require special counseling. Confidentiality and sensitivity are important[19].

7. Research and Ethics

Research raises several ethical issues which should be taken into consideration:

- ➢ There should be no misuse of the information discovered
- ➢ Responsibility for protecting the participant's data result should be maintained[20]
- ➢ The privacy, anonymity and rights of the persons involved in the research project should be protected and respected[20]

Regarding research publications, some significant issues include:

- ➢ All teams involved in the process of publication including the author, expert reviewer and members of journal editorial boards must respect the integrity and privacy of each other[21].
- ➢ The editorial review process should be unbiased and must contribute to the quality control; it is an essential step to maintain the originality of the research.
- ➢ Authorship addresses the individuals involved in the research project and the final publication. It must ensure clearly who may claim a right to authorship and in which order the authors should be listed[22].

Pledge to the Profession

It would be an ethically good practice if the technical medical laboratory staff would take an obligation towards their profession.

American Society for Clinical Laboratory Science's pledge for laboratory practice is a good example of how professional laboratory staff must follow[1].

"As a clinical laboratory professional, I strive to:

- Maintain and promote standards of excellence in performing and advancing the art and science of my profession
- Preserve the dignity and privacy of others
- Uphold and maintain the dignity and respect of our profession
- Seek to establish cooperative and respectful working relationships with other health professionals
- Contribute to the general well-being of the community
- I will actively demonstrate my commitment to these responsibilities throughout my professional life"

REFERENCES

1. The American Society for Clinical Laboratory Science. Code of Ethics. Available at: http://www.ascls.org/about-us/code-of-ethics. Accessed in March 2015.
2. Farnell LR. Greek Hero Cults and Ideas of Immortality; The Gifford Lectures: Delivered in the University of St. Andrews in the Year 1920. Whitefish, Montana: Kessinger Publishing, 2004: 269.
3. Rutkow IM. Surgery: An Illustrated History. St. Louis: Mosby-Year Book, 1993: 27.
4. Rogers WA, Draper H. Confidentiality and the Ethics of Medical Ethics. J Med Ethics 2003; 29(4):220-4.
5. Appel JM. Must My Doctor Tell My Partner? Rethinking Confidentiality in the HIV Era. Med Health R I 2006; 89(6):223-4.
6. Guidance on Professional Conduct for Nursing and Midwifery Students. Nursing and Midwifery Council. http://www.city.ac.uk/__data/assets/pdf_file/0007/65536/Guidance-on-Professional-

Conduct-for-Nursing-and-Midwifery-Students.pdf. Accessed in March 2015.
7. Code of Ethics | ASCLS. The Code of Ethics of the American Society for Clinical Laboratory Science. www.ascls.org/about-us/code-of-ethics. Accessed in March 2015.
8. Shahangian S, Snyder SR. Laboratory Medicine Quality Indicators: A Review of the Literature. Am J Clin Pathol 2009; 131(3):418-31.
9. Baur X, Budnik LT, Ruff K, et al. Ethics, Morality, and Conflicting Interests: How Questionable Professional Integrity in Some Scientists Supports Global Corporate Influence in Public Health. Int J Occup Environ Health 2015; 37(1):172-5.
10. General Medical Council. Standards and Ethics Guidance for Doctors. http://www.gmc-uk.org/publications/standards_guidance_for_doctors.asp. Accessed in March 2015.
11. Wade D. Ethics of Collecting and Using Healthcare Data. BMJ 2007; 334(7608):1330-1.
12. Gunter TD, Nicolas PT. The Emergence of National Electronic Health Record Architectures in the United States and Australia: Models, Costs, and Questions. J Med Internet Res 2005; 7(1):e[3].
13. US Department of Health & Human Services. Health Information Privacy. Available at: www.hhs.gov/ocr/privacy. Accessed in March 2015.
14. Policy on the Verbal Reporting of Critical Value Results, KHUH, Policy number LAB0006, effective from April 2014. IBMS publications www.ibms.org/publications.
15. Schäfer D, Baumann R, Kettner M. Ethics and Reproductive Medicine. Hum Reprod Update 1996; 2(5):447-56.
16. Tierney E, Ebrahim W, Baithun S, et al. Is It Time for a Virtual Autopsy Service in Bahrain? Bahrain Med Bull 2014; 36(4): 211-3.
17. International Society of Blood Transfusion during the Society's 16th Congress.
Available at: www.sciencedirect.com/science/article/pii/S0887 796393700279. Accessed in March 2015.
18. Grainger B, Margolese E, Partington E. Legal and Ethical Considerations in Blood Transfusion. CMAJ 1997; 156(11):S50-54.
19. Boyd KM. HIV Infection and AIDS: The Ethics of Medical Confidentiality. J Med Ethics 1992; 18(4):173-9.

20. Shaw SE, Petchey RP, Chapman J, et al. A Double-Edged Sword? Health Research and Research Governance in UK Primary Care. Soc Sci Med 2009; 68(5):912-8.
21. Chanson H. Research Quality, Publications and Impact in Civil Engineering into the 21st Century. Publish or Perish, Commercial versus Open Access, Internet versus Libraries? Canadian Journal of Civil Engineering 2007; 34(8): 946-51.
22. Chanson H. Digital Publishing, Ethics and Hydraulic Engineering: The Elusive or "Boring" Bore? In: Stefano Pagliara 2nd International Junior Researcher and Engineer Workshop on Hydraulic Structures (IJREW'08), Pisa, Italy, 2008: 3-13.

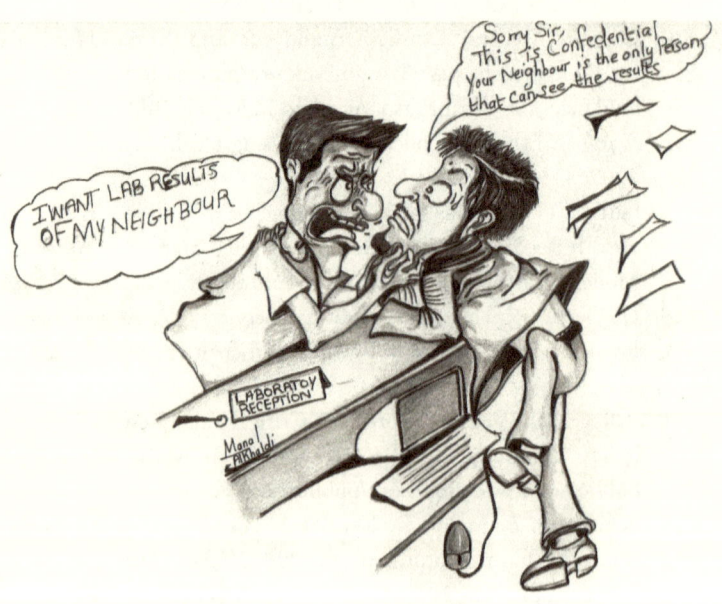

VISION OF THE FUTURE KING HAMAD UNIVERSITY HOSPITAL RESEARCH CENTER

Jaffar M Albareeq

It is proposed that the Research Center occupies the top floor of the Oncology Center; the main offices and laboratories are as follows: (a facility for future laboratories should be provided 8,000–10,000 square ft.)

1. Research Administration Offices

2. Data Analysis Laboratory (staffed by statisticians and computer analysts)

3. Online search, teleconference facility and training laboratory accommodating 50 at a time

4. Diabetic and Obesity Unit
    Metabolic Cell Biology Laboratory with the facility for

    a. Metabolic signaling and disease
    b. Clinical research facility
    c. Rodents metabolic and behavioral testing laboratory
    d. Nutrition, metabolism and diabetes laboratory

5. **Pediatric Unit**

    a. Sickle cell, thalassemia and autism genetics laboratory
    b. Autism laboratory and behavioral therapy laboratory
    c. Type 1 diabetes laboratory
    d. Genetic disease, muscle development, regeneration and RNA biology laboratory

6. **Stem Cell Research Unit**

    a. Cord blood storage facility
    b. Inherited diseases laboratory
    c. Stem cell laboratory therapy
    d. Genome project studies laboratory
    e. Gene therapy laboratory
    f. Pharmacogenetic laboratory

7. **Immunology and Allergy Laboratory**

8. **Cancer Unit**

    a. Cancer genetic laboratory
    b. Molecular cancer laboratory
    c. Cancer biomarker laboratory
    d. Stem cell and chemotherapy
    e. Research facility for apoptosis and cell death research, tumor development and tumor microenvironment

9. **Molecular Unit**

    a. DNA, RNA and cellular enzymes laboratory and facilities for polymerase chain reaction (PCR), gel electrophoresis, Macromolecule blotting and probing, Southern blotting, Northern blotting, Western blotting and Eastern blotting
    b. Organ cloning laboratory

10. **Neuroscience and Aging Unit**

    a. Degenerative disease
    b. Development and aging

11. **Infectious and Inflammatory Diseases**

    a. Infectious diseases laboratory
    b. Inflammatory diseases laboratory
    c. Inflammatory biomarker laboratory

12. **Assisted Reproduction Technology Unit**

    a. Storage of semen for ten years
    b. Storage of female ova for 15 years
    c. Storage of embryos
    d. Gametes, zygote and embryo research laboratory
    e. Nuclear transfer or cloning
    f. Ovary and Uterus physiology laboratory

13. **Bone Marrow Transplant Laboratory**

14. **Ophthalmology Unit**

    a. Corneal graft bank
    b. Retinal stem cell therapy

Staffing

A. **Scientist Researchers:** These researchers have PhDs, MDs or both and devote at least 50 percent of their time to research. All scientists are also professors at RCSI or AGU and many are active physicians at KHUH. Scientists generally holding peer-reviewed research grants and work with a team of graduate students, postdoctoral fellows, technicians and coordinators.

B. **Associate Researchers:** These are physicians, nurses or other healthcare professionals who devote between 25 and 50 percent of their time to clinical research.
C. **Clinical Researchers:** These are physicians, nurses or other healthcare professionals who devote between 5 and 25 percent of their time to clinical research.
D. **Affiliate Researchers:** These are researchers who have primary affiliations with other institutions, but maintain significant collaborations with KHUH or have some research funding administered by KHUH.
E. **Trainee Clinical Researchers:** These are researchers recruited from various clinical disciplines and trained in research methodology for 3-4 weeks.

The Research and Ethics Committee considers the Belmont Report as an applicable document to any research performed at King Hamad University Hospital

BASIC PRINCIPLES OF THE BELMONT REPORT[1]

In the Nuremberg war crime trials after World War II, Nazi biomedical researchers were prosecuted for their abuses against prisoners in concentration camps. A proper set of standards for judging the physicians and scientists who had conducted experiments on the prisoners was drawn up by the presiding international tribunal. The basic ethics of the Nuremberg Code continues to serve as a cornerstone for modern regulations regarding the use of human participants in experimentation. **Its principles emphasize a profound respect for the voluntary nature of research participation, the idea of true informed consent and the personal ethical responsibilities of the investigator to ensure human welfare.**

In 1979, the Belmont Report stated that "Ethical Principles and Guidelines for the Protection of Human Subjects of Research" was published in the United States to provide a succinct description of the mandate for review of research involving human research participants. Regulation and guidelines concerning the use of human research participants in the U.S., and increasingly so in other countries, are based on the following fundamental elements excerpted from the Belmont Report:

Respect for Persons has at least two ethical considerations. The individual human research participant is treated as an autonomous being—a person who makes decisions or deliberates about personal goals and then acts upon them. Those persons who are not able to make and carry out decisions for themselves, such as children or sick people or those who have a mental disorder must be protected from coercion by others and from activities that harm them. How much protection needed is related to the risk and likelihood of benefit. **In research, respect for persons demands that participants enter into a research program voluntarily and with good information about the research goals.**

Beneficence has to do with doing good to the individual. In the Belmont Report, beneficence is understood in a stronger sense, as an obligation, such as to do no harm and to "maximize possible benefits and minimize possible harms" to the individual research participant. "Do no harm" is a Hippocratic principle of medical ethics though its extension into research implies that "one should not injure one person regardless of the benefits that might come to others." Although sometimes you could not know that something is harmful until you try it and in the process of trying or experimentation, persons may be exposed to the risk of harm. The Hippocratic Oath also requires that physicians benefit patients "according to their best judgment," but, again, learning what would benefit may mean exposing a person to risk.

The principle of beneficence obligates both society and the individual investigator. Society has to give forethought to the long-term benefits and risks that result from increased knowledge and the development of new therapeutic devices or procedures that are the outcome of research. **Investigators and their institutions have to plan to maximize benefits and minimize risks.**

Justice, in this report, refers to the benefits and harms to individual subjects of research. In the 19th and early 20th century hospitals in America, the burdens of experimentation fell upon the poor charity patients while the rewards of the improved medical care went primarily to the rich private patients. The Nazi researchers and concentration camp prisoners provide another good example of injustice. The benefits and burdens of research should be justly distributed. The selection of research participants needs to be constantly monitored to determine whether some pools of participants are systematically selected from simply because they are easily available or vulnerable or easy to manipulate, rather than chosen for reasons directly related to the research problem being studied.

Applications for Comprehensive Ethical Principles in Research Involving Human Participants

Informed Consent

A critical component of respecting human participants is the **informed consent process**. The consent document is a written summary of the information that should be provided to the participant. Many investigators use it as a guide for the verbal explanation of the study. The participant's signature on the form shows agreement to participate in a study, but that is only one part of the consent process. The entire informed consent process involves:

1. Giving a participant adequate information about the study
2. Providing adequate opportunity for the participant to consider all options, responding to the participant's questions
3. Ensuring that the participant has comprehended this information
4. Obtaining the participant's voluntary agreement to participate
5. Continuing to provide information as the participant or situation requires

In the case of subjects whose ability to understand might be limited, such as children, mentally disabled patients or those who are very ill, special provision may have to be made. With these groups, permission must frequently be sought from a third party who would be in a position to understand the incompetent participant's situation and act in their best interest. This third person should be able to follow the research and be able to withdraw the participant if it appears to be in the best interest of the individual.

To summarize: the informed consent process must allow human participants, as much as they are able, to be given the opportunity to choose what would or would not happen to them. The consent process must include information to the participant about the research; the participant must understand the information and volunteer rather than be coerced into participation.

Assessment of Risks and Benefits

Assessing risks and benefits means the researcher needs to assemble all data that explains why the research would obtain the benefits that are sought by the research project. The review committee of the researcher's sponsoring institution, upon review of the collected data, could decide whether the risks to the subjects are justified. The prospective participant could determine whether or not to participate.

The term "risk" refers to the possibility that harm might occur. There are many kinds of risks, such as psychological, physical, legal, social and economic hardship. The term "benefit" in the research context refers to something positive as related to health or welfare. Risks and benefits affect not only individual participants, but also their families and society at large. Importantly, in the past regulations about human subjects, **the risk to participants has been outweighed by the sum of both the anticipated benefit to participants and the anticipated benefit to society in the form of new knowledge to be gained by the research.**

Selection of Participants

The principle of justice—that benefits and risks of research be distributed fairly. Researchers are not just if they only select disadvantaged persons for risky research or only provide beneficial research to groups they favor. Special classes of injustice arise when participants are drawn from vulnerable populations, like those institutionalized or incarcerated in prisons, racial minorities, economically disadvantaged or the very sick.

Table 1: Basic Ethical Principles and Applications as Outlined in the Belmont Report

Ethical Principles for Research	Applications of Ethical Principles for Research
Respect for Persons Individuals should be treated as autonomous agents. Persons with diminished autonomy are entitled to protection.	**Informed Consent** Volunteer research participants, to the degree that they are capable, must be given the opportunity to choose what shall or shall not happen to them. The consent process must include three elements: • Information • Comprehension • Voluntary participation
Beneficence Human participants should not be harmed. Research should maximize possible benefits and minimize possible risks.	**Assessment of Risks and Benefits** The nature and scope of risks and benefits must be assessed in a systematic way.
Justice The benefits and risks of research must be distributed fairly.	**Selection of Participants** There must be fair procedures and outcomes in the selection of research participants.

REFERENCE

1. http://www.hhs.gov/ohrp/humansubjects/guidance/belmont.html. Accessed on 8 July 2015.

Uniform Requirements for Manuscripts Submitted to Biomedical Journals

King Hamad University Hospital recommends that researchers/authors abide by Recommendations for the Conduct, Reporting, Editing, and Publication of Scholarly Work in Medical Journals Updated December 2016.

http://www.icmje.org/icmje-recommendations.pdf

www.ingramcontent.com/pod-product-compliance
Lightning Source LLC
Chambersburg PA
CBHW030922180526
45163CB00002B/436